D0948235

Critical Care and Cardiac Medicine

Current Clinical Strategies

2006 Edition

Matthew Brenner, MD
Associate Professor of Medicine
Pulmonary and Critical Care Division
University of California, Irvine

Georgina Heal, MD
Ryan M. Klein, MD
Scott T. Gallacher, MD
Guy Foster, MD
Michael Krutzik, MD

Farhad Mazdisnian, MD
Roham T. Zamanian, MD
Hans Poggemeyer, MD
H. L. Daneschvar, MD
S. E. Wilson, MD

Division of Pulmonary and Critical Care Medicine
College of Medicine
University of California, Irvine

Current Clinical Strategies Publishing

www.ccspublishing.com/ccs

Digital Book and Updates

Purchasers of this book may download the digital book and updates for Palm, Pocket PC, Windows and Macintosh. The digital books can be downloaded at the Current Clinical Strategies Publishing Internet site:

www.ccspublishing.com/ccs/cc.htm.

Current Clinical Strategies Publishing

www.ccspublishing.com/ccs

27071 Cabot Road
Laguna Hills, California 92653
Phone: 800-331-8227
E-Mail: info@ccspublishing.com

Printed in USA   ISBN 1-929622-72-4

Contents

Advanced Cardiac Life Support

EMERGENCY CARDIAC CARE

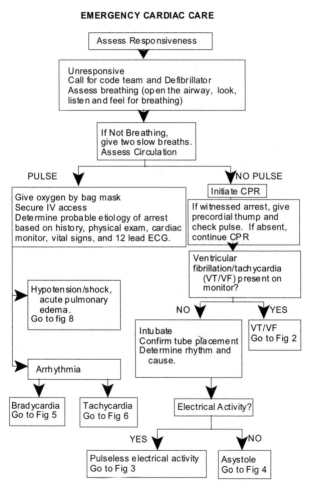

Fig 1 - Algorithm for Adult Emergency Cardiac Care

**VENTRICULAR FIBRILLATION AND PULSELESS
VENTRICULAR TACHYCARDIA**

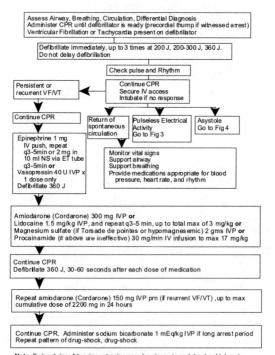

Assess Airway, Breathing, Circulation, Differential Diagnosis
Administer CPR until defibrillator is ready (precordial thump if witnessed arrest)
Ventricular Fibrillation or Tachycardia present on defibrillator

Defibrillate immediately, up to 3 times at 200 J, 200-300 J, 360 J.
Do not delay defibrillation

Check pulse and Rhythm

Persistent or
recurrent VF/VT

Continue CPR
Secure IV access
Intubate if no response

Continue CPR

Return of
spontaneous
circulation

Pulseless Electrical
Activity
Go to Fig 3

Asystole
Go to Fig 4

Epinephrine 1 mg
 IV push, repeat
 q3-5min or 2 mg in
 10 ml NS via ET tube
 q3-5min or
Vasopressin 40 U IVP x
 1 dose only
Defibrillate 360 J

Monitor vital signs
Support airway
Support breathing
Provide medications appropriate for blood
 pressure, heart rate, and rhythm

Amiodarone (Cordarone) 300 mg IVP or
Lidocaine 1.5 mg/kg IVP, and repeat q3-5 min, up to total max of 3 mg/kg or
Magnesium sulfate (if Torsade de pointes or hypomagnesemic) 2 gms IVP or
Procainamide (if above are ineffective) 30 mg/min IV infusion to max 17 mg/kg

Continue CPR
Defibrillate 360 J, 30-60 seconds after each dose of medication

Repeat amiodarone (Cordarone) 150 mg IVP prn (if reurrent VF/VT) , up to max
cumulative dose of 2200 mg in 24 hours

Continue CPR. Administer sodium bicarbonate 1 mEq/kg IVP if long arrest period
Repeat pattern of drug-shock, drug-shock

Note: Epinephrine, lidocaine, atropine may be given via endotracheal tube at
2-2.5 times the IV dose. Dilute in 10 cc of saline.
After each intravenous dose, give 20-30 mL bolus of IV fluid and elevate
extremity.

Fig 2 - Ventricular Fibrillation and Pulseless Ventricular Tachycardia

PULSELESS ELECTRICAL ACTIVITY

Pulseless Electrical Activity Includes:
        Electromechanical dissociation (EMD)
        Pseudo-EMD
        Idioventricular rhythms
        Ventricular escape rhythms
        Bradyasystolic rhythms
        Postdefibrillation idioventricular rhythms

Initiate CPR, secure IV access, intubate, assess pulse.

Determine differential diagnosis and treat underlying cause:
  Hypoxia (ventilate)
  Hypovolemia (infuse volume)
  Pericardial tamponade (perform pericardiocentesis)
  Tension pneumothorax (perform needle decompression)
  Pulmonary embolism (thrombectomy, thrombolytics)
  Drug overdose with tricydics, digoxin, beta, or calcium blockers
  Hyperkalemia or hypokalemia
  Acidosis (give bicarbonate)
  Myocardial infarction (thrombolytics)
  Hypothermia (active rewarming)

Epinephrine 1.0 mg IV bolus q3-5 min, or high dose
    epinephrine 0.1 mg/kg IV push q3-5 min; may give via
    ET tube.
Continue CPR

If bradycardia (<60 beats/min), give atropine 1 mg IV, q3-5
    min, up to total of 0.04 mg/kg
Consider bicarbonate, 1 mEq/kg IV (1-2 amp, 44 mEq/amp),
    if hyperkalemia or other indications.

Fig 3 - Pulseless Electrical Activity

ASYSTOLE

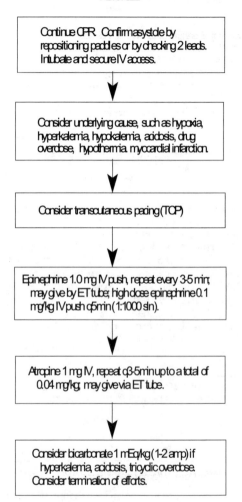

Continue CPR. Confirm asystole by repositioning paddles or by checking 2 leads. Intubate and secure IV access.

Consider underlying cause, such as hypoxia, hyperkalemia, hypokalemia, acidosis, drug overdose, hypothermia, myocardial infarction.

Consider transcutaneous pacing (TCP)

Epinephrine 1.0 mg IV push, repeat every 3-5 min; may give by ET tube; high dose epinephrine 0.1 mg/kg IV push q5min (1:1000 sln).

Atropine 1 mg IV, repeat q3-5min up to a total of 0.04 mg/kg; may give via ET tube.

Consider bicarbonate 1 mEq/kg (1-2 amp) if hyperkalemia, acidosis, tricyclic overdose. Consider termination of efforts.

Fig 4 - Asystole

BRADYCARDIA

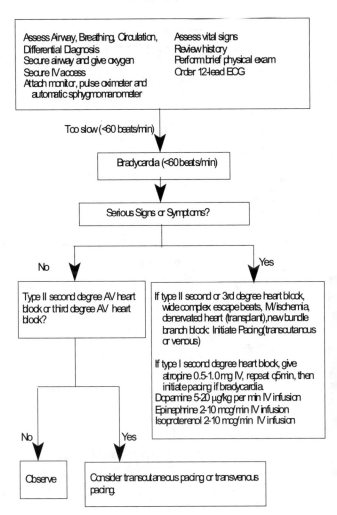

Assess Airway, Breathing, Circulation, Differential Diagnosis
Secure airway and give oxygen
Secure IV access
Attach monitor, pulse oximeter and automatic sphygmomanometer

Assess vital signs
Review history
Perform brief physical exam
Order 12-lead ECG

Too slow (<60 beats/min)

Bradycardia (<60 beats/min)

Serious Signs or Symptoms?

No

Yes

Type II second degree AV heart block or third degree AV heart block?

If type II second or 3rd degree heart block, wide complex escape beats, MI/ischemia, denervated heart (transplant), new bundle branch block: Initiate Pacing(transcutaneous or venous)

If type I second degree heart block, give atropine 0.5-1.0 mg IV, repeat q5min, then initiate pacing if bradycardia.
Dopamine 5-20 µg/kg per min IV infusion
Epinephrine 2-10 mcg/min IV infusion
Isoproterenol 2-10 mcg/min IV infusion

No

Yes

Observe

Consider transcutaneous pacing or transvenous pacing.

Fig 5 - Bradycardia (with patient not in cardiac arrest).

TACHYCARDIA

Assess Airway, Breathing, Circulation, Differential Diagnosis
Assess Vitals, Secure Airway
Review history and examine patient
Give 100% oxygen, secure IV access.
Attach ECG monitor, pulse oximeter, blood pressure monitor.
Order 12-lead ECG, portable chest x-ray.

UNSTABLE with serious signs or symptoms?
Unstable includes, hypotension, heart failure, chest pain, myocardial infarction, decreased mental status, dyspnea

Yes →

IMMEDIATE CARDIOVERSION
Atrial flutter 50 J, paroxysmal supraventricular tachycardia 50 J, atrial fibrillation 100 J, monomorphic ventricular tachycardia100 J, polymorphic V tach 200 J. Premedicate with midazolam (Versed) 2-5 mg IVP when possible.

No or borderline →

Torsade de pointes (polymorphic VT)

→ Correct underlying cause: Hypokalemia, drug overdose (tricyclic, phenothiazine, antiarrhythmic class Ia, Ic, III)) →

Ventricular tachycardia (VT)

→ Amiodarone 150-300 mg IV over 10-20 min →

Wide-complex tachycardia of uncertain type

→ If uncertain if V tach, give Adenosine 6 mg rapid IV push over 1-3 sec

→ Adenosine 12 mg, rapid IV push over 1-3 sec (may repeat once in 1-2 min) →

1-2 min

Paroxysmal supraventricular narrow complex tachycardia (PSVT)

→ Vagal maneuvers: Carotid sinus massage if no bruits

→ Adenosine 6 mg, rapid IV push over 1-3 sec →

1-2 min

Atrial fibrillation Atrial flutter

→ Determine Etiology: Hypoxia, ischemia, MI, pulmonary embolus, hyperthyroidism, electrolyte abnormality, theophylline, inotropes.

→ Control Rate: Diltiazem, verapamil, digoxin esmolol, metoprolol

→ Cardioversion of atrial fibrillation to sinus rhythm: If less than 2 days and rate controlled: Procainamide or amiodarone, followed by cardioversion.
If more than 2 days: Coumadin for 3 weeks; control rate, start antiarrhythmic agent, then electrical cardioversion.

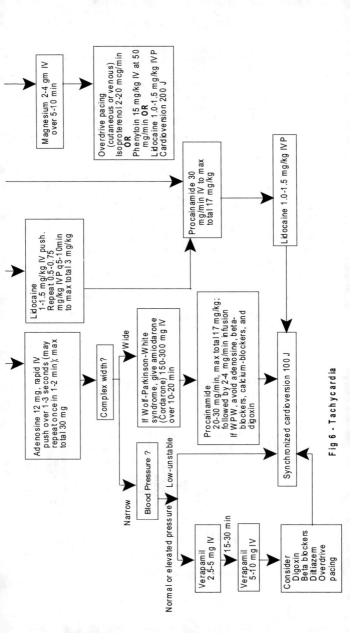

Magnesium 2-4 gm IV over 5-10 min

Overdrive pacing (cutaneous or venous)
Isoproterenol 2-20 mcg/min
OR
Phenytoin 15 mg/kg IV at 50 mg/min **OR**
Lidocaine 1.0-1.5 mg/kg IVP
Cardioversion 200 J

Lidocaine 1-1.5 mg/kg IV push.
Repeat 0.5-0.75 mg/kg IVP q5-10min
to max total 3 mg/kg

Procainamide 30 mg/min IV to max total 117 mg/kg

Lidocaine 1.0-1.5 mg/kg IVP

Adenosine 12 mg, rapid IV push over 1-3 seconds (may repeat once in 1-2 min); max total 30 mg

Complex width?

Wide

If Wolf-Parkinson-White syndrome, give amiodarone (Cordarone) 150-300 mg IV over 10-20 min

Procainamide 20-30 mg/min, max total 17 mg/kg; followed by 2-4 mg/min infusion
If WPW, avoid adenosine, beta-blockers, calcium-blockers, and digoxin

Narrow

Blood Pressure ?

Low-unstable

Normal or elevated pressure

Verapamil 2.5-5 mg IV

15-30 min

Verapamil 5-10 mg IV

Consider
Digoxin
Beta blockers
Diltiazem
Overdrive pacing

Synchronized cardioversion 100 J

Fig 6 - Tachycardia

STABLE TACHYCARDIA

Stable tachycardia with serious signs and symptoms related to the tachycardia. Patient not in cardiac arrest.

If ventricular rate is >150 beats/min, prepare for immediate cardioversion.
Treatment of Stable Patients is based on Arrhythmia Type:

Ventricular Tachycardia:
  Procainamide (Pronestyl) 30 mg/min IV, up to a total max of 17 mg/kg, or
  Amiodarone (Cordarone) 150-300 mg IV over 10-20 min, or
  Lidocaine 0.75 mg/kg. Procainamide should be avoided if ejection fraction is <40%.

Paroxysmal Supraventricular Tachycardia: Carotid sinus pressure (if bruits absent), then adenosine 6 mg rapid IVP, followed by 12 mg rapid IVP x 2 doses to max total 30 mg. If no response, verapamil 2.5-5.0 mg IVP; may repeat dose with 5-10 mg IVP if adequate blood pressure; or Esmolol 500 mcg/kg IV over 1 min, then 50 mcg/kg/min IV infusion, and titrate up to 200 mcg/kg/min IV infusion.

Atrial Fibrillation/Flutter:
  Ejection fraction ≥40%: Diltiazem (Cardiazem) 0.25 mg/kg IV over 2 min; may repeat 0.35 mg/kg IV over 2 min prn x 1 to control rate. Then give procainamide (Pronestyl) 30 mg/min IV infusion, up to a total max of 17 mg/kg
  Ejection fraction <40%: Digoxin 0.5 mg IVP, then 0.25 mg IVP q4h x 2 to control rate. Then give amiodarone (Cordarone) 150-300 mg IV over 10-20 min.

Check oxygen saturation, suction device, intubation equipment. Secure IV access

Premedicate whenever possible with Midazolam (Versed) 2-5 mg IVP or sodium pentothal 2 mg/kg rapid IVP

Synchronized cardioversion
Atrial flutter	50 J
PSVT	50 J
Atrial	100 J
Monomorphic V-tach	100 J
Polymorphic V tach	200 J

Fig 7 - Stable Tachycardia (not in cardiac arrest)

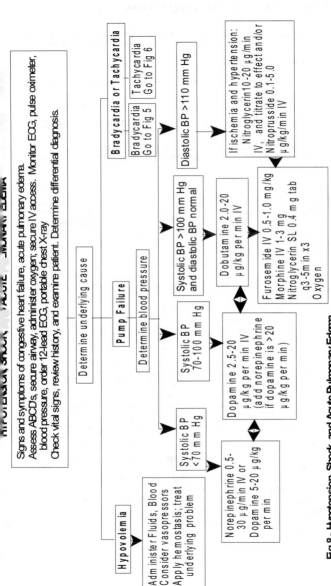

HYPOTENSION, SHOCK, AND ACUTE PULMONARY EDEMA

Signs and symptoms of congestive heart failure, acute pulmonary edema.
Assess ABCDs; secure airway, administer oxygen; secure IV access. Monitor ECG, pulse oximeter, blood pressure; order 12-lead ECG, portable chest X-ray.
Check vital signs, review history, and examine patient. Determine differential diagnosis.

Determine underlying cause

Hypovolemia

Administer Fluids, Blood
Consider vasopressors
Apply hemostasis; treat underlying problem

Pump Failure

Determine blood pressure

Systolic BP <70 mm Hg

Norepinephrine 0.5-30 μg/min IV or Dopamine 5-20 μg/kg per min

Systolic BP 70-100 mm Hg

Dopamine 2.5-20 μg/kg per min IV (add norepinephrine if dopamine is >20 μg/kg per min)

Systolic BP >100 mm Hg and diastolic BP normal

Dobutamine 2.0-20 μg/kg per min IV

Furosemide IV 0.5-1.0 mg/kg
Morphine IV 1-3 mg
Nitroglycerin SL 0.4 mg tab q3-5 min x3
Oxygen

Bradycardia or Tachycardia

Bradycardia
Go to Fig 5

Tachycardia
Go to Fig 6

Diastolic BP >110 mm Hg

If ischemia and hypertension:
Nitroglycerin 10-20 μg/min IV, and titrate to effect and/or
Nitroprusside 0.1-5.0 μg/kg/min IV

Fig 8 - Hypotension, Shock, and Acute Pulmonary Edema

Critical and Cardiac Care Patient Management

T. Scott Gallacher, MD, MS

Critical Care History and Physical Examination

Chief complaint: Reason for admission to the ICU.

History of present illness: This section should included pertinent chronological events leading up to the hospitalization. It should include events during hospitalization and eventual admission to the ICU.

Prior cardiac history: Angina (stable, unstable, changes in frequency), exacerbating factors (exertional, rest angina). History of myocardial infarction, heart failure, coronary artery bypass graft surgery, angioplasty. Previous exercise treadmill testing, ECHO, ejection fraction. Request old ECG, ECHO, impedance cardiography, stress test results, and angiographic studies.

Chest pain characteristics:
A. **Pain:** Quality of pain, pressure, squeezing, tightness
B. **Onset of pain:** Exertional, awakening from sleep, relationship to activities of daily living (ADLs), such as eating, walking, bathing, and grooming.
C. **Severity and quality:** Pressure, tightness, sharp, pleuritic
D. **Radiation:** Arm, jaw, shoulder
E. **Associated symptoms:** Diaphoresis, dyspnea, back pain, GI symptoms.
F. **Duration:** Minutes, hours, days.
G. **Relieving factors:** Nitroclycerine, rest.

Cardiac risk factors: Age, male, diabetes, hypercholesteremia, low HDL, hypertension, smoking, previous coronary artery disease, family history of arteriosclerosis (eg, myocardial infarction in males less than 50 years old, stroke).

Congestive heart failure symptoms: Orthopnea (number of pillows), paroxysmal nocturnal dyspnea, dyspnea on exertional, edema.

Peripheral vascular disease symptoms: Claudication, transient ischemic attack, cerebral vascular accident.

COPD exacerbation symptoms: Shortness of breath, fever, chills, wheezing, sputum production, hemoptysis (quantify), corticosteroid use, previous intubation.

Past medical history: Peptic ulcer disease, renal disease, diabetes, COPD. Functional status prior to hospitalization.

Medications: Dose and frequency. Use of nitroglycerine, beta-agonist, steroids.

Allergies: Penicillin, contrast dye, aspirin; describe the specific reaction (eg, anaphylaxis, wheezing, rash, hypotension).

Social history: Tobacco use, alcohol consumption, intravenous drug use.

Review of systems: Review symptoms related to each organ system.

Critical Care Physical Examination

Vital signs:
   Temperature, pulse, respiratory rate, BP (vital signs should be given in ranges)
   Input/Output: IV fluid volume/urine output.
   Special parameters: Oxygen saturation, pulmonary artery wedge pressure (PAWP), systemic vascular resistance (SVR), ventilator settings, impedance cardiography.
General: Mental status, Glasgow coma score, degree of distress.
HEENT: PERRLA, EOMI, carotid pulse.
Lungs: Inspection, percussion, auscultation for wheezes, crackles.
Cardiac: Lateral displacement of point of maximal impulse; irregular rate,, irregular rhythm (atrial fibrillation); S3 gallop (LV dilation), S4 (myocardial infarction), holosystolic apex murmur (mitral regurgitation).
Cardiac murmurs: 1/6 = faint; 2/6 = clear; 3/6 = loud; 4/6 = palpable; 5/6 = heard with stethoscope off the chest; 6/6 = heard without stethoscope.
Abdomen: Bowel sounds normoactive, abdomen soft and nontender.
Extremities: Cyanosis, clubbing, edema, peripheral pulses 2+.
Skin: Capillary refill, skin turgor.
Neuro
   Deficits in strength, sensation.
   Deep tendon reflexes: 0 = absent; 1 = diminished; 2 = normal; 3 = brisk; 4 = hyperactive clonus.
   Motor Strength: 0 = no contractility; 1 = contractility but no joint motion; 2 = motion without gravity; 3 = motion against gravity; 4 = motion against some resistance; 5 = motion against full resistance (normal).
Labs: CBC, INR/PTT; chem 7, chem 12, Mg, pH/pCO_2/pO_2. CXR, ECG, impedance cardiography, other diagnostic studies.

Impression/Problem list: Discuss diagnosis and plan for each problem by system.
Neurologic Problems: List and discuss neurologic problems
Pulmonary Problems: Ventilator management.
Cardiac Problems: Arrhythmia, chest pain, angina.
GI Problems: H2 blockers, nasogastric tubes, nutrition.
Genitourinary Problems: Fluid status: IV fluids, electrolyte therapy.
Renal Problems: Check BUN, creatinine. Monitor fluids and electrolytes. Monitor inputs and outputs.
Hematologic Problems: Blood or blood products, DVT prophylaxis, check hematocrit/hemoglobin.
Infectious Disease: Plans for antibiotic therapy; antibiotic day number, culture results.
Endocrine/Nutrition: Serum glucose control, parenteral or enteral nutrition, diet.

Admission Check List

1. **Call and request** old chart, ECG, and x-rays.
2. **Stat labs:** CBC, chem 7, cardiac enzymes (myoglobin, troponin, CPK), INR, PTT, C&S, ABG, UA, cardiac enzymes (myoglobin, troponin, CPK).
3. **Labs:** Toxicology screens and drug levels.
4. **Cultures:** Blood culture x 2, urine and sputum culture (before initiating

antibiotics), sputum Gram stain, urinalysis.
5. **CXR, ECG**, diagnostic studies.
6. **Discuss case with resident, attending**, and family.

Critical Care Progress Note

ICU Day Number:
Antibiotic Day Number:
Subjective: Patient is awake and alert. Note any events that occurred overnight.
Objective: Temperature, maximum temperature, pulse, respiratory rate, BP, 24-hr input and output, pulmonary artery pressure, pulmonary capillary wedge pressure, cardiac output.
Lungs: Clear bilaterally
Cardiac: Regular rate and rhythm, no murmur, no rubs.
Abdomen: Bowel sounds normoactive, soft-nontender.
Neuro: No local deficits in strength, sensation.
Extremities: No cyanosis, clubbing, edema, peripheral pulses 2+.
Labs: CBC, ABG, chem 7.
ECG: **Chest x-ray:**
Impression and Plan: Give an overall impression, and then discuss impression and plan by organ system:
  Cardiovascular:
  Pulmonary:
  Neurological:
  Gastrointestinal:
  Renal:
  Infectious:
  Endocrine:
  Nutrition:

Procedure Note

A procedure note should be written in the chart when a procedure is performed. Procedure notes are brief operative notes.

Procedure Note

Date and time:
Procedure:
Indications:
Patient Consent: Document that the indications, risks and alternatives to the procedure were explained to the patient. Note that the patient was given the opportunity to ask questions and that the patient consented to the procedure in writing.
Lab tests: Relevant labs, such as the INR and CBC
Anesthesia: Local with 2% lidocaine
Description of Procedure: Briefly describe the procedure, including sterile prep, anesthesia method, patient position, devices used, anatomic location of procedure, and outcome.
Complications and Estimated Blood Loss (EBL):
Disposition: Describe how the patient tolerated the procedure.
Specimens: Describe any specimens obtained and labs tests which were ordered.
Name of Physician: Name of person performing procedure and supervising staff.

Discharge Note

The discharge note should be written in the patient's chart prior to discharge.

Discharge Note

Date/time:
Diagnoses:
Treatment: Briefly describe treatment provided during hospitalization, including surgical procedures and antibiotic therapy.
Studies Performed: Electrocardiograms, CT scans, CXR.
Discharge Medications:
Follow-up Arrangements:

Fluids and Electrolytes

Maintenance Fluids Guidelines:
　　70 kg Adult: D5 1/4 NS with KCl 20 mEq/Liter at 125 mL/hr.
Specific Replacement Fluids for Specific Losses:
　　Gastric (nasogastric tube, emesis): D5 1/2 NS with KCL 20 mEq/L.
　　Diarrhea: D5LR with KCl 15 mEq/liter. Provide 1 liter of replacement for each 1 kg or 2.2 lb of body weight lost.

Bile: D5LR with sodium bicarbonate 25 mEq/liter (1/2 amp).
Pancreatic: D5LR with sodium bicarbonate 50 mEq/liter (1 amp).

Blood Component Therapy

A. **Packed red blood cells (PRBCs).** Each unit provides 250-400 cc of volume, and each unit should raise hemoglobin by 1 gm/dL and hematocrit by 3%. PRBCs are usually requested in two unit increments.

B. **Type and screen.** Blood is tested for A, B, Rh antigens, and antibodies to donor erythrocytes. If blood products are required, the blood can be rapidly prepared by the blood bank. O negative blood is used when type and screen information is not available, but the need for transfusion is emergent.

C. **Type and cross match** sets aside specific units of packed donor red blood cells. If blood is needed on an urgent basis, type and cross should be requested.

D. **Platelets.** Indicated for bleeding if there is thrombocytopenia or platelet dysfunction in the setting of uncontrolled bleeding. Each unit of platelet concentrate should raise the platelet count by 5,000-10,000. Platelets are usually transfused 6-10 units at a time, which should increase the platelet count by 40-60,000. Thrombocytopenia is defined as a platelet count of less than 60,000. For surgery, the count should be greater than 50,000.

E. **Fresh Frozen Plasma (FFP)** is used for active bleeding secondary to liver disease, warfarin overdose, dilutional coagulopathy secondary to multiple blood transfusions, disseminated intravascular coagulopathy, and vitamin K and coagulation factor deficiencies. Administration of FFP requires ABO typing, but not cross matching.
  1. Each unit contains coagulation factors in normal concentration.
  2. Two to four units are usually required for therapeutic intervention.

F. **Cryoprecipitate**
  1. Indicated in patients with Hemophilia A, Von Willebrand's disease, and any state of hypofibrinogenemia requiring replacement (DIC), or reversal of thrombolytic therapy.
  2. Cryoprecipitate contains factor VIII, fibrinogen, and Von Willebrand factor. The goal of therapy is to maintain the fibrinogen level above 100 mL/dL, which is usually achieved with 10 units given over 3-5 minutes.

Central Parenteral Nutrition

Infuse 40-50 mL/hr of amino acid dextrose solution in the first 24 hr; increase daily by 40 mL/hr increments until providing 1.3-2 x basal energy requirement and 1.2-1.7 gm protein/kg/d (see formula, page 169)

Standard Solution per Liter

Amino acid solution (Aminosyn) 7-10%	500 mL
Dextrose 40-70%	500 mL
Sodium	35 mEq
Potassium	36 mEq
Chloride	35 mEq
Calcium	4.5 mEq
Phosphate	9 mMol
Magnesium	8.0 mEq
Acetate	82-104 mEq
Multi-Trace Element Formula	1 mL/d
Regular insulin (if indicated)	10-20 U/L
Multivitamin 12 (2 amp)	10 mL/d
Vitamin K (in solution, SQ, IM)	10 mg/week
Vitamin B 12	1000 mcg/week

Fat Emulsion:
-Intralipid 20% 500 mL/d IVPB infused in parallel with standard solution at 1 mL/min x 15 min; if no adverse reactions, increase to 20-50 mL/hr. Serum triglyceride level should be checked 6h after end of infusion (maintain <250 mg/dL).

Cyclic Total Parenteral Nutrition
-12-hour night schedule; taper continuous infusion in morning by reducing rate to half original rate for 1 hour. Further reduce rate by half for an additional hour, then discontinue. Restart TPN in evening. Taper at beginning and end of cycle. Final rate should be 185 mL/hr for 9-10h with 2 hours of taper at each end, for total of 2000 mL.

Peripheral Parenteral Supplementation
-Amino acid solution (ProCalamine) 3% up to 3 L/d at 125 cc/h OR
-Combine 500 mL amino acid solution 7% or 10% (Aminosyn) and 500 mL 20% dextrose and electrolyte additive. Infuse at up to 100 cc/hr in parallel with intralipid 10% or 20% at 1 mL/min for 15 min (test dose); if no adverse reactions, infuse 500 mL/d at 20 mL/hr.

Special Medications
-Famotidine (Pepcid) 20 mg IV q12h or 40 mg/day in TPN **OR**
-Ranitidine (Zantac) 50 mg IV q6-8h.
-Insulin sliding scale or continuous IV infusion.

Labs
   Baseline: Draw labs below. Chest x-ray, plain film for tube placement
   Daily Labs: Chem 7, osmolality, CBC, cholesterol, triglyceride (6h after end of infusion), serum phosphate, magnesium, calcium, urine specific gravity.
   Weekly Labs: Protein, iron, TIBC, INR/PTT, 24h urine nitrogen and creatinine. Pre-albumin, transferrin, albumin, total protein, AST, ALT, GGT, alkaline phosphatase, LDH, amylase, total bilirubin.

Enteral Nutrition

General Measures: Daily weights, nasoduodenal feeding tube. Head of bed at 30 degrees while enteral feeding and 2 hours after completion. Record bowel movements.

Continuous Enteral Infusion: Initial enteral solution (Osmolite, Pulmocare, Jevity) 30 mL/hr. Measure residual volume q1h x 12h, then tid; hold feeding for 1 h if residual is more than 100 mL of residual. Increase rate by 25-50 mL/hr at 24 hr intervals as tolerated until final rate of 50-100 mL/hr (1 cal/mL) as tolerated. Three tablespoons of protein powder (Promix) may be added to each 500 cc of solution. Flush tube with 100 cc water q8h.

Enteral Bolus Feeding: Give 50-100 mL of enteral solution (Osmolite, Pulmocare, Jevity) q3h initially. Increase amount in 50 mL steps to max of 250-300 mL q3-4h; 30 kcal of nonprotein calories/d and 1.5 gm protein/kg/d. Before each feeding measure residual volume, and delay feeding by 1 h if >100 mL. Flush tube with 100 cc of water after each bolus.

Special Medications:
-Metoclopramide (Reglan) 10-20 mg PO, IM, IV, or in J tube q6h.
-Famotidine (Pepcid) 20 mg J-tube q12h **OR**
-Ranitidine (Zantac) 150 mg in J-tube bid.

Symptomatic Medications:
-Loperamide (Imodium) 24 mg PO or in J-tube q6h, max 16 mg/d prn **OR**
-Diphenoxylate/atropine (Lomotil) 5-10 mL (2.5 mg/5 mL) PO or in J-tube q4-6h, max 12 tabs/d **OR**
-Kaopectate 30 cc PO or in J-tube q6h.

Radiographic Evaluation of Common Interventions

I. **Central intravenous lines**
   A. **Central venous catheters** should be located well above the right atrium, and not in a neck vein. Rule out pneumothorax by checking that the lung markings extend completely to the rib cages on both sides. Examine for hydropericardium ("water bottle" sign, mediastinal widening).
   B. **Pulmonary artery catheter tips** should be located centrally and posteriorly, and not more than 3-5 cm from midline.
II. **Endotracheal tubes.** Verify that the tube is located 3 cm below the vocal cords and 2-4cm above the carina; the tip of tube should be at the level of aortic arch.
III. **Tracheostomies.** Verify by chest x-ray that the tube is located halfway between the stoma and the carina; the tube should be parallel to the long axis of the trachea. The tube should be approximately 2/3 of width of the trachea; the cuff should not cause bulging of the trachea walls. Check for subcutaneous air in the neck tissue and for mediastinal widening secondary to air leakage.
IV. **Nasogastric tubes and feeding tubes.** Verify that the tube is in the stomach and not coiled in the esophagus or trachea. The tip of the tube should not be near the gastroesophageal junction.
V. **Chest tubes.** A chest tube for pneumothorax drainage should be near the level of the third intercostal space. If the tube is intended to drain a free-flowing pleural effusion, it should be located inferior-posteriorly, at or about the level of the eighth intercostal space. Verify that the side port of the tube is within the thorax.
VI. **Mechanical ventilation.** Obtain a chest x-ray to rule out pneumothorax, subcutaneous emphysema, pneumomediastinum, or subpleural air cysts. Lung infiltrates or atelectasis may diminish or disappear after initiation of mechanical ventilation because of increased aeration of the affected lung lobe.

Arterial Line Placement

Procedure
1. Obtain a 20-gauge 1 1/2-2 inch catheter over needle assembly (Angiocath), arterial line setup (transducer, tubing and pressure bag containing heparinized saline), arm board, sterile dressing, lidocaine, 3 cc syringe, 25-gauge needle, and 3-O silk suture.
2. The radial artery is the most frequently used artery. Use the Allen test to verify the patency of the radial and ulnar arteries. Place the extremity on an arm board with a gauze roll behind the wrist to maintain hyperextension.
3. Prep the skin with povidone-iodine and drape; infiltrate 1% lidocaine using a 25-gauge needle. Choose a site where the artery is most superficial and distal.
4. Palpate the artery with the left hand, and advance the catheter-over-needle assembly into the artery at a 30-degree angle to the skin. When a flash of blood is seen, hold the needle in place and advance the catheter into the artery. Occlude the artery with manual pressure while the pressure tubing is connected.

5. Advance the guide wire into the artery, and pass the catheter over the guide wire. Suture the catheter in place with 3-0 silk and apply dressing.

Central Venous Catheterization

I. **Indications for central venous catheter cannulation:** Monitoring of central venous pressures in shock or heart failure; management of fluid status; insertion of a transvenous pacemaker; administration of total parenteral nutrition; administration of vesicants (chemotherapeutic agents).

II. **Location:** The internal jugular approach is relatively contraindicated in patients with a carotid bruit, stenosis, or an aneurysm. The subclavian approach has an increased risk of pneumothorax in patients with emphysema or bullae. The external jugular or internal jugular approach is preferable in patients with coagulopathy or thrombocytopenia because of the ease of external compression. In patients with unilateral lung pathology or a chest tube already in place, the catheter should be placed on the side of predominant pathology or on the side with the chest tube if present.

III. **Technique for insertion of external jugular vein catheter**
1. The external jugular vein extends from the angle of the mandible to behind the middle of the clavicle, where it joins with the subclavian vein. Place the patient in Trendelenburg's position. Cleanse skin with Betadine-iodine solution, and, using sterile technique, inject 1% lidocaine to produce a skin weal. Apply digital pressure to the external jugular vein above the clavicle to distend the vein.
2. With a 16-gauge thin wall needle, advance the needle into the vein. Then pass a J-guide wire through the needle; the wire should advance without resistance. Remove the needle, maintaining control over the guide wire at all times. Nick the skin with a No. 11 scalpel blade.
3. With the guide wire in place, pass the central catheter over the wire and remove the guide wire after the catheter is in place. Cover the catheter hub with a finger to prevent air embolization.
4. Attach a syringe to the catheter hub and ensure that there is free backflow of dark venous blood. Attach the catheter to an intravenous infusion.
5. Secure the catheter in place with 2-0 silk suture and tape. The catheter should be replaced weekly or if there is any sign of infection.
6. Obtain a chest x-ray to confirm position and rule out pneumothorax.

IV. **Internal jugular vein cannulation.** The internal jugular vein is positioned behind the stemocleidomastoid muscle lateral to the carotid artery. The catheter should be placed at a location at the upper confluence of the two bellies of the stemocleidomastoid, at the level of the cricoid cartilage.
1. Place the patient in Trendelenburg's position and turn the patient's head to the contralateral side.
2. Choose a location on the right or left. If lung function is symmetrical and no chest tubes are in place, the right side is preferred because of the direct path to the superior vena cava. Prepare the skin with Betadine solution using sterile technique and place a drape. Infiltrate the skin and deeper tissues with 1% lidocaine.
3. Palpate the carotid artery. Using a 22-gauge scout needle and syringe, direct the needle lateral to the carotid artery towards the ipsilateral nipple at a 30-degree angle to the neck. While aspirating, advance the needle until the vein is located and blood flows back into the syringe.

4. Remove the scout needle and advance a 16-gauge, thin wall catheter-over-needle with an attached syringe along the same path as the scout needle. When back flow of blood is noted into the syringe, advance the catheter into the vein. Remove the needle and confirm back flow of blood through the catheter and into the syringe. Remove the syringe, and use a finger to cover the catheter hub to prevent air embolization.

5. With the 16-gauge catheter in position, advance a 0.89 mm x 45 cm spring guide wire through the catheter. The guidewire should advance easily without resistance.

6. With the guidewire in position, remove the catheter and use a No. 11 scalpel blade to nick the skin.

7. Place the central vein catheter over the wire, holding the wire secure at all times. Pass the catheter into the vein, remove the guidewire, and suture the catheter with 0 silk suture, tape, and connect it to an IV infusion.

8. Obtain a chest x-ray to rule out pneumothorax and confirm position of the catheter.

V. Subclavian vein cannulation. The subclavian vein is located in the angle formed by the medial ⅓ of the clavicle and the first rib.

1. Position the patient supine with a rolled towel located between the patient's scapulae, and turn the patient's head towards the contralateral side. Prepare the area with Betadine iodine solution, and, using sterile technique, drape the area and infiltrate 1% lidocaine into the skin and tissues.

2. Advance the 16-gauge catheter-over-needle, with syringe attached, into a location inferior to the mid-point of the clavicle, until the clavicle bone and needle come in contact.

3. Slowly probe down with the needle until the needle slips under the clavicle, and advance it slowly towards the vein until the catheter needle enters the vein and a back flow of venous blood enters the syringe. Remove the syringe, and cover the catheter hub with a finger to prevent air embolization.

4. With the 16-gauge catheter in position, advance a 0.89 mm x 45 cm spring guide wire through the catheter. The guide wire should advance easily without resistance.

5. With the guide wire in position, remove the catheter, and use a No. 11 scalpel blade to nick the skin.

6. Place the central line catheter over the wire, holding the wire secure at all times. Pass the catheter into the vein, and suture the catheter with 2-0 silk suture, tape, and connect to an IV infusion.

7. Obtain a chest x-ray to confirm position and rule out pneumothorax.

VI. Pulmonary artery catheterization procedure

A. Using sterile technique, cannulate a vein using the technique above. The subclavian vein or internal jugular vein is commonly used.

B. Advance a guide wire through the cannula, then remove the cannula, but leave the guide wire in place. Keep the guide wire under control at all times. Nick the skin with a number 11 scalpel blade adjacent to the guide wire, and pass a number 8 French introducer over the wire into the vein. Remove the wire and connect the introducer to an IV fluid infusion, and suture with 2-0 silk.

C. Pass the proximal end of the pulmonary artery catheter (Swan Ganz) to an assistant for connection to a continuous flush transducer system.

D. Flush the distal and proximal ports with heparin solution, remove all bubbles, and check balloon integrity by inflating 2 cc of air. Check the pressure transducer by quickly moving the distal tip and watching the monitor for response.

E. Pass the catheter through the introducer into the vein, then inflate the balloon with 1.0 cc of air, and advance the catheter until the balloon is in or near the right atrium.

F. The approximate distance to the entrance of the right atrium is determined from the site of insertion:
Right internal jugular vein: 10-15 cm.
Subclavian vein: 10 cm.
Femoral vein: 35.45 cm.

G. Advance the inflated balloon, while monitoring pressures and wave forms as the PA catheter is advanced. Advance the catheter through the right ventricle into the main pulmonary artery until the catheter enters a distal branch of the pulmonary artery and is stopped (as evidenced by a pulmonary wedge pressure waveform).

H. Do not advance the catheter while the balloon is deflated, and do not withdraw the catheter with the balloon inflated. After placement, obtain a chest X-ray to ensure that the tip of catheter is no farther than 3-5 cm from the mid-line, and no pneumothorax is present.

Normal Pulmonary Artery Catheter Values

Right atrial pressure	1-7 mm Hg
RVP systolic	15-25 mm Hg
RVP diastolic	8-15 mm Hg
Pulmonary artery pressure	
PAP systolic	15-25 mm Hg
PAP diastolic	8-15 mm Hg
PAP mean	10-20 mm Hg

Cardiovascular Disorders

Roham T. Zamanian, MD
Farhad Mazdisnian, MD
Michael Krutzik, MD

Acute Coronary Syndromes (ST-Segment Elevation MI, Non-ST-Segment Elevation MI, and Unstable Angina)

Acute myocardial infarction (AMI) and unstable angina are part of a spectrum known as the acute coronary syndromes (ACS), which have in common a ruptured atheromatous plaque. Plaque rupture results in platelet activation, adhesion, and aggregation, leading to partial or total occlusion of the artery.

These syndromes include ST-segment elevation MI, non-ST-segment elevation MI, and unstable angina. The ECG presentation of ACS includes ST-segment elevation infarction, ST-segment depression (including non–Q-wave MI and unstable angina), and nondiagnostic ST-segment and T-wave abnormalities. Patients with ST-segment elevation MI require immediate reperfusion, mechanically or pharmacologically. The clinical presentation of myocardial ischemia is most often acute chest pain or discomfort.

I. Characteristics of chest pain and associated symptoms

  A. **Ischemic chest pain** can be characterized by the the OPQRST mnemonic. Symptoms associated with the highest relative risk of myocardial infarction (MI) include radiation to an upper extremity, particularly when there is radiation to both arms, and pain associated with diaphoresis or with nausea and vomiting. The patient should be asked if current pain is reminiscent of prior MI.

   1. **Onset.** Ischemic pain is typically gradual in onset, although the intensity of the discomfort may wax and wane.

   2. **Provocation and palliation.** Ischemic pain is generally provoked by an activity. Ischemic pain does not change with respiration or position. It may or may not respond to nitroglycerin.

   3. **Quality.** Ischemic pain is often characterized more as a discomfort than pain, and it may be difficult to describe. The patient may describe the pain as squeezing, tightness, pressure, constriction, crushing, strangling, burning, heartburn, fullness in the chest, band-like sensation, knot in the center of the chest, lump in throat, ache, heavy weight on chest. It is usually not described as sharp, fleeting, knife-like, stabbing, or pins and needles-like. The patient may place his clenched fist in the center of the chest, which is known as the "Levine sign."

   4. **Radiation.** Ischemic pain often radiates to other parts of the body including the upper abdomen (epigastrium), shoulders, arms (upper and forearm), wrist, fingers, neck and throat, lower jaw and teeth (but not upper jaw), and not infrequently to the back (specifically the interscapular region). Pain radiating to the upper extremities is highly suggestive of ischemic pain.

5. **Site.** Ischemic pain is not felt in one specific spot, but rather it is a diffuse discomfort that may be difficult to localize. The patient often indicates the entire chest, rather than localizing it to a specific area by pointing a single finger.

6. **Time course.** Angina is usually brief (two to five minutes) and is relieved by rest or with nitroglycerin. In comparison, patients with an acute coronary syndrome (ACS) may have chest pain at rest, and the duration is variable but generally lasts longer than 30 minutes. Classic anginal pain lasting more than 20 minutes is particularly suggestive of an ACS.

7. **Associated symptoms.** Ischemic pain is often associated with shortness of breath, which may reflect pulmonary congestion. Other symptoms may include belching, nausea, indigestion, vomiting, diaphoresis, dizziness, lightheadedness, clamminess, and fatigue. Elderly women and diabetics are more likely to present with such "atypical" symptoms in lieu of classic chest pain.

B. **Characteristics of nonischemic chest discomfort:**
1. Pleuritic pain, sharp or knife-like pain related to respiratory movements or cough.
2. Primary or sole location in the mid or lower abdominal region.
3. Any discomfort localized with one finger.
4. Any discomfort reproduced by movement or palpation.
5. Constant pain lasting for days.
6. Fleeting pains lasting for a few seconds or less.
7. Pain radiating into the lower extremities or above the mandible.

C. Some patients with ACS present with atypical types of chest pain. Acute ischemia is diagnosed in 22 percent of patients who present with sharp or stabbing pain and 13 percent who presented with pleuritic-type pain.

D. **Atypical symptoms.** Some patients with acute coronary syndrome (ACS) present with atypical symptoms rather than chest pain. One-third have no chest pain on presentation to the hospital. These patients often present with symptoms such as dyspnea alone, nausea and/or vomiting, palpitations, syncope, or cardiac arrest. They are more likely to be older, diabetic, and women.

E. **Additional history and exam**
1. **Historical features increasing likelihood of ACS**
   a. Patients with a prior history of coronary heart disease (CHD) have a significantly increased risk of recurrent ischemic events.
   b. A prior history of other vascular disease is associated with a risk of cardiac ischemic events comparable to that seen with a prior history of CHD.
   c. Risk factors for CHD, including especially age, sex, diabetes, hypertension, hyperlipidemia, and cigarette smoking.
   d. Recent cocaine use.
2. **Focused physical exam**
   a. Responsiveness, airway, breathing and circulation.
   b. Evidence of systemic hypoperfusion (hypotension; tachycardia; impaired cognition; cool, clammy, pale, ashen skin). Cardiogenic shock complicating acute MI requires aggressive evaluation and management.
   c. Ventricular arrhythmias. Sustained ventricular tachyarrhythmias in the periinfarction period must be treated immediately because of their deleterious effect on cardiac output, possible exacerbation of myocardial ischemia, and the risk of deterioration into VF.

    d. Evidence of heart failure (jugular venous distention, rales, S3 gallop, hypotension, tachycardia).

    e. A screening neurologic examination should be performed to assess for focal lesions or cognitive deficits that might preclude safe use of thrombolytic therapy.

Differential diagnosis of severe or prolonged chest pain

Myocardial infarction
Unstable angina
Aortic dissection
Gastrointestinal disease (esophagitis, esophageal spasm, peptic ulcer disease, biliary colic, pancreatitis)
Pericarditis
Chest-wall pain (musculoskeletal or neurologic)
Pulmonary disease (pulmonary embolism, pneumonia, pleurisy, pneumothorax)
Psychogenic hyperventilation syndrome

---

    f. Exam findings increasing likelihood of MI. Findings on physical examination associated with significantly increased risk of myocardial infarction are hypotension (systolic blood pressure <80) and signs of pump failure (ie, new or worsening pulmonary crackles, new S3, new or worsening MR murmur).

II. Immediate management

  A. During the initial assessment phase, the following steps should be accomplished for any patient with significant risk of ACS:

    1. Airway, breathing, and circulation assessed

    2. 12-lead ECG obtained

    3. Resuscitation equipment brought nearby

    4. Cardiac monitor attached

    5. Oxygen given

    6. IV access and blood work obtained

    7. Aspirin 162 to 325 mg given

    8. Nitrates and morphine given (unless contraindicated)

  B. Twelve-lead ECG should be obtained in all patients with possible coronary ischemia. The 12-lead ECG provides the basis for initial diagnosis and management. The initial ECG is often not diagnostic in patients with ACS. The ECG should be repeated at 5 to 10 minute intervals, if the initial ECG is not diagnostic but the patient remains symptomatic and there is a high clinical suspicion for MI.

  C. Cardiac monitoring should be initiated with emergency resuscitation equipment (including a defibrillator and airway equipment) nearby.

  D. Supplemental oxygen should be initiated to maintain oxygen saturation above 90 percent.

  E. Intravenous access should be established, with blood drawn for initial laboratory work, including cardiac biomarkers.

  F. Aspirin should be given to all patients at a dose of 162 to 325 mg to chew and swallow, unless there is a compelling contraindication (eg, history of anaphylactic reaction) or it has been taken prior to presentation.

  G. Sublingual nitroglycerin should be administered at a dose of 0.4 mg every five minutes for a total of three doses, after which an assessment should be made about the need for intravenous nitroglycerin. Before this is done, all men should be questioned about the use of sildenafil (Viagra), vardenafil (Levitra), or tadalafil (Cialis); nitrates are contraindicated if these drugs have been used in the last 24 hours (36 hours with tadalafil) because of the risk of severe hypotension.

1. Extreme care should also be taken before giving nitrates in the setting of an inferior myocardial infarction with possible involvement of the right ventricle. Nitrate use can cause severe hypotension in this setting.

H. **Intravenous morphine sulfate** at an initial dose of 2 to 4 mg, with increments of 2 to 8 mg, repeated at 5 to 15 minute intervals, should be given for the relief of chest pain and anxiety.

III. **ECG-based management of the Four major ischemic syndromes**

A. ST elevation (Q wave) MI is manifested by Q waves that are usually preceded by hyperacute T waves and ST elevations, and followed by T wave inversions. Clinically significant ST segment elevation is considered to be present if it is greater than 1 mm (0.1 mV) in at least two anatomically contiguous leads.

B. Non-ST elevation (Non-Q wave) MI is manifested by ST depressions or T-wave inversions without Q waves.

C. Noninfarction subendocardial ischemia (classic angina), manifested by transient ST segment depressions.

D. Noninfarction transmural ischemia (Prinzmetal's variant angina) is manifested by transient ST segment elevations or paradoxical T wave normalization.

E. **Localization of ischemia.** The anatomic location of a transmural infarct is determined by which ECG leads show ST elevation and/or increased T wave positivity:

1. Acute transmural anterior wall ischemia - one or more of the precordial leads (V1-V6)
2. Anteroseptal ischemia - leads V1 to V3
3. Apical or lateral ischemia - leads aVL and I, and leads V4 to V6
4. Inferior wall ischemia - leads II, III, and aVF
5. Right ventricular ischemia - right-sided precordial leads

F. The right-sided leads V4R, V5R, and V6R should be obtained if there is evidence of inferior wall ischemia, demonstrated by ST elevation in leads II, III, and aVF. The posterior leads V7, V8, and V9 may also be helpful if there is evidence of posterior wall ischemia, as suggested by prominent R waves and ST depressions in leads V1 and V2.

G. **Serial ECGs.** The initial ECG is often not diagnostic in patients with ACS. Therefore, if the initial ECG is not diagnostic, but the patient remains symptomatic and there is a high clinical suspicion for MI, it is recommended that the ECG be repeated at 5 to 10 minute intervals.

H. **LBBB or pacing.** Both LBBB, which is present in 7 percent of patients with an acute MI, and pacing can interfere with the electrocardiographic diagnosis of coronary ischemia. Careful evaluation of the ECG may show some evidence of ACS in patients with these abnormalities. The clinical history and cardiac enzymes are of primary importance in diagnosing an ACS in this setting.

I. **ST elevation.** Regardless of the presence or absence of Q waves, an ST elevation MI (STEMI) is diagnosed in the following circumstances:

1. ST segment elevation >1 mm is present in two or more anatomically contiguous leads.
2. The elevations are considered to represent ischemia and not pericarditis or left ventricular aneurysm.

J. The patient should also be presumed to have an acute STEMI if the ECG shows a left bundle branch block that is not known to be old and the clinical suspicion for an ACS is high.

K. Reperfusion therapy. A patient with an acute STEMI should undergo reperfusion therapy with either primary percutaneous intervention (PCI) or thrombolysis, if less than 12 hours has elapsed from the onset of symptoms. Benefit from thrombolysis is significantly greater when given within four hours of the onset of symptoms. Primary PCI is preferred to thrombolysis when readily available.

L. Antiplatelet therapy is indicated in all patients with STEMI, regardless of whether they undergo reperfusion therapy, unless an absolute contraindication exists.

    1. Aspirin is the preferred antiplatelet agent and should be given in a dose of 162 to 325 mg to chew and swallow as soon as possible to any patient with STEMI.

    2. Clopidogrel (Plavix) is recommended in all patients treated with primary PCI and stenting. A 600 mg loading dose should begin in these patients, and primary PCI should be done within 90 minutes. Benefit from the use of clopidogrel in addition to aspirin has been demonstrated in patients under 75 years of age undergoing thrombolysis. Patients over 75 years of age generally receive 75 mg because of the increased risk of hemorrhage.

    3. Clopidogrel (300 mg loading dose followed by 75 mg once daily) is given to patients who are managed without reperfusion therapy in this setting based upon the benefit demonstrated in nonrevascularized patients with non-ST elevation syndromes.

    4. Clopidogrel can also be given in the rare case where aspirin is contraindicated.

M. Glycoprotein IIb/IIIa inhibitors. Treatment with abciximab should be started as early as possible prior to PCI, with or without stent, in patients with STEMI.

N. Beta blockers should be administered to all patients with ST elevation MI without contraindications. Early intravenous use of a cardioselective agent, such as metoprolol or atenolol, is recommended:

    1. Intravenous metoprolol can be given in 5 mg increments by slow intravenous administration (5 mg over one to two minutes), repeated every five minutes for a total initial dose of 15 mg. Patients who tolerate this regimen should then receive oral therapy beginning 15 minutes after the last intravenous dose (25 to 50 mg every six hours for 48 hours) followed by a maintenance dose of 100 mg twice daily.

    2. Intravenous atenolol can be given in a 5 mg dose, followed by another 5 mg, five minutes later. Patients who tolerate this regimen should then receive oral therapy beginning one to two hours after the last intravenous dose (50 to 100 mg/day).

    3. Esmolol (Brevibloc) (50 mcg/kg per min increasing to a maximum of 200 to 300 mcg/kg per min) can be used if an ultrashort acting beta blocker is required.

O. Intravenous nitroglycerin can be given for treatment of persistent pain, congestive heart failure, or hypertension, provided there are no contraindications (eg, use of drugs for erectile dysfunction or right ventricular infarction). The goal of therapy is a 10 percent reduction in the systolic blood pressure or a 30 percent reduction in hypertensive patients.

Therapy for Non-ST Segment Myocardial Infarction and Unstable Angina	
Treatment	**Recommendations**
Antiplatelet agent	Aspirin, 325 mg (chewable)
Nitrates	Sublingual nitroglycerin (Nitrostat), one tablet every 5 min for total of three tablets initially, followed by IV form (Nitro-Bid IV, Tridil) if needed
Beta-blocker	• IV therapy recommended for prompt response, followed by oral therapy. • Metoprolol (Lopressor), 5 mg IV every 5 min for three doses • Atenolol (Tenormin) 5 mg IV q5min x 2 doses • Esmolol (Brevibloc), initial IV dose of 50 micrograms/kg/min and adjust up to 200-300 micrograms/kg/min
Heparin	80 U/kg IVP, followed by 15 U/kg/hr. Goal: aPTT 50-70 sec
Enoxaparin (Lovenox)	1 mg/kg IV, followed by 1 mg/kg subcutaneously bid
Glycoprotein IIb/IIIa inhibitors	Eptifibatide (Integrilin) or tirofiban (Aggrastat) for patients with high-risk features in whom an early invasive approach is planned
Adenosine diphosphate receptor-inhibitor	Consider clopidogrel (Plavix) therapy, 300 mg x 1, then 75 mg qd.
Cardiac catheterization	Consideration of early invasive approach in patients at intermediate to high risk and those in whom conservative management has failed

P. Potassium. The ACC/AHA guidelines recommend maintaining the serum potassium concentration above 4.0 meq/L in an acute MI. Maintaining a serum magnesium concentration above 2.0 meq/L is recommended.

Q. Unfractionated heparin (UFH) is given to patients with with STEMI undergoing percutaneous or surgical revascularization, and to patients undergoing thrombolysis with selective fibrinolytic agents. Low molecular weight heparin (LMWH) is an alternative to UFH in patients receiving thrombolysis provided they are younger than 75 years of age and have no renal dysfunction.

Treatment Recommendations for ST-Segment Myocardial Infarction

Supportive Care for Chest Pain
· All patients should receive supplemental oxygen, 2 L/min by nasal canula, for a minimum of three hours
· Two large-bore IVs should be placed

Aspirin:

Inclusion	Clinical symptoms or suspicion of AMI
Exclusion	Aspirin allergy, active GI bleeding
Recommendation	Chew and swallow one dose of160-325 mg, then orally qd

Thrombolytics:

Inclusion	All patients with ischemic pain and ST-segment elevation (≥ 1 mm in ≥ 2 contiguous leads) within 6 hours of onset of persistent pain, age <75 years. All patients with a new bundle branch block and history suggesting acute MI.
Exclusion	Active internal bleeding; history of cerebrovascular accident; recent intracranial or intraspinal surgery or trauma; intracranial neoplasm, arteriovenous malformation, or aneurysm; known bleeding diathesis; severe uncontrolled hypertension
Recommendation	**Reteplase (Retavase)** 10 U IVP over 2 min x 2. Give second dose of 10 U 30 min after first dose **OR** **Tenecteplase (TNKase):** <60 kg: 30 mg IVP; 60-69 kg: 35 mg IVP; 70-79 kg: 40 mg IVP; 80-89 kg: 45 mg IVP; $\geq$90 kg: 50 mg IVP **OR** **t-PA (Alteplase, Activase)** 15 mg IV over 2 minutes, then 0.75 mg/kg (max 50 mg) IV over 30 min, followed by 0.5 mg/kg (max 35 mg) IV over 30 min.

Heparin:

Inclusion	**Administer concurrently with thrombolysis**
Exclusion	Active internal or CNS bleeding
Recommendation	Heparin 60 U/kg (max 4000 U) IVP, followed by 12 U/kg/hr (max 1000 U/h) continuous IV infusion x 48 hours. Maintain aPTT 50-70 seconds

Beta-Blockade:

Inclusion	All patients with the diagnosis of AMI. Begin within 12 hours of diagnosis of AMI
Exclusion	Severe COPD, hypotension, bradycardia, AV block, pulmonary edema, cardiogenic shock
Recommendation	Metoprolol (Lopressor), 5 mg IV push every 5 minutes for three doses; followed by 25 mg PO bid. Titrate up to 100 mg PO bid **OR** Atenolol (Tenormin), 5 mg IV, repeated in 5 minutes, followed by 50-100 mg PO qd.

Nitrates:	
Inclusion	All patients with ischemic-type chest pain
Exclusion	Hypotension; caution in right ventricular infarction
Recommendation	0.4 mg NTG initially q 5 minutes, up to 3 doses or nitroglycerine aerosol, 1 spray sublingually every 5 minutes. IV infusion of NTG at 10-20 mcg/min, titrating upward by 5-10 mcg/min q 5-10 minutes (max 3 mcg/kg/min). Slow or stop infusion if systolic BP <90 mm Hg

ACE-Inhibitors or Angiotensin Receptor Blockers:	
Inclusion	All patients with the diagnosis of AMI. Initiate treatment within 24 hours after AMI
Exclusion	Bilateral renal artery stenosis, angioedema caused by previous treatment
Recommendation	Lisinopril (Prinivil) 2.5-5 mg qd, titrate to 10-20 mg qd. Maintain systolic BP >100 mmHg or Valsartan (Diovan) 40 mg bid, titrate to 160 mg bid

IV. **Non-ST elevation.** Patients with coronary ischemia but who do not manifest ST elevations on ECG are considered to have unstable angina (UA) or a non-ST elevation myocardial infarction (NSTEMI). UA and NSTEMI comprise part of the spectrum of ACS.
  A. Angina is considered unstable if it presents in any of the following three ways:
    1. Rest angina, generally lasting longer than 20 minutes
    2. New onset angina that markedly limits physical activity
    3. Increasing angina that is more frequent, lasts longer, or occurs with less exertion than previous angina
  B. NSTEMI is distinguished from UA by the presence of elevated serum biomarkers. ST segment elevations and Q waves are absent in both UA and NSTEMI. Unstable angina and NSTEMI are frequently indistinguishable initially because an elevation in serum biomarkers is usually not detectable for four to six hours after an MI, and at least 12 hours are required to detect elevations in all patients.
  C. **Risk stratification**
    1. The TIMI investigators developed a 7-point risk stratification tool that predicted the risk of death, reinfarction, or urgent revascularization at 14 days after presentation. This scoring system includes the following elements:
      a. Age >65.
      b. Three or more cardiac risk factors.
      c. Aspirin use in the preceding seven days.
      d. Two or more anginal events in the preceding 24 hours.
      e. ST-segment deviation on presenting ECG.
      f. Increased cardiac biomarkers.
      g. Prior coronary artery stenosis >50 percent.
    2. Patients are considered to be high risk if they have a TIMI risk score of 5 or greater (one point is given for each element) and low risk if the score is 2 or below.
    3. Additional factors associated with death and reinfarction at 30 days after presentation include:

      a. Bradycardia or tachycardia

      b. Hypotension

      c. Signs of heart failure (new or worsening rales, MR murmur, S3 gallop)

      d. Sustained ventricular tachycardia

D. Reperfusion. Thrombolytic therapy should not be administered to patients with UA or NSTEMI unless subsequent ECG monitoring documents ST segment elevations that persist. An aggressive approach to reperfusion using PCI is best suited for patients with a TIMI risk score $\geq$5 or possibly other high-risk features.

E. Antiplatelet therapy is a cornerstone of treatment in UA and NSTEMI.

  1. Aspirin is the preferred antiplatelet agent and should be given to all patients with suspected ACS.

  2. Clopidogrel (300-600 mg) is indicted in patients undergoing PCI. A class IIa recommendation was given to their use in patients with high-risk features in whom PCI is not planned.

F. Beta-blocker, nitroglycerin, morphine. The use of these agents in NSTEMI is similar to that in STEMI.

G. Electrolyte repletion. Low electrolytes, particularly potassium and magnesium, which are associated with an increased risk of ventricular fibrillation in the setting of ACS, should be replaced.

H. Heparin. The ACC/AHA guidelines recommend the use of enoxaparin in preference to unfractionated heparin in patients with UA/NSTEMI, provided there is no evidence of renal failure and CABG is not planned within 24 hours.

I. Disposition of NSTEMI

  1. High-risk patients have a high-risk ACS if ST segment depression ($\geq$0.05 mV [0.5 mm]) is present in two or more contiguous leads and/or the TIMI risk score is $\geq$5. This patient is admitted to an intensive care unit, coronary care unit, or monitored cardiac unit depending upon the persistence of symptoms and evidence of hemodynamic compromise. Those with persistent pain or hemodynamic compromise generally undergo urgent angiography and revascularization. Others with resolution of symptoms and stable hemodynamics are typically referred for early elective angiography and revascularization if appropriate.

      a. If there is no ST segment elevation or depression or new LBBB, regardless of the presence or absence of Q waves, the patient with definite or probable ACS should still be admitted to a monitored care unit for further evaluation. Those patients manifesting high-risk features either on presentation or during their emergency room course should be considered for early PCI.

  2. Moderate-risk patient. Patients who have no ECG changes and are at moderate risk for ACS can be admitted to a chest pain observation unit, if available, for further evaluation because a small percentage (2 to 4 percent) will have an ACS.

  3. Low-risk patient. Patients with no ECG changes, a TIMI risk score below 3, and no other concerning features in their presentation can be considered for early provocative testing or possible discharge with outpatient follow-up. Patients at very low risk in whom there is clear objective evidence for a non-ischemic cause of their chest pain can be discharged with outpatient follow-up.

V. Cardiac biomarkers (enzymes). Serial serum biomarkers (also called cardiac enzymes) of acute myocardial damage, such as troponin T and I, creatine kinase (CK)-MB, and myoglobin, are essential for confirming the diagnosis of infarction. The most commonly used are troponin T or I and CK-MB, which can be measured by rapid bedside assay.

A. **Sensitivity and specificity**. An elevation in the serum concentration of one or more of the above markers is seen in virtually all patients with an acute MI. However, the sensitivity of these tests is relatively low until four to six hours after symptom onset. Thus, a negative test in this time period does not exclude infarction. Furthermore, some patients do not show a biomarker elevation for as long as 12 hours.

B. Therefore, in patients who have an acute STEMI, reperfusion therapy should not await the results of cardiac biomarkers. In patients without diagnostic ST segment elevation, serial biomarker testing is performed after four or more hours if the initial values are indeterminate, the ECG remains nondiagnostic, and clinical suspicion remains high.

Common Markers for Acute Myocardial Infarction			
Marker	Initial Elevation After MI	Mean Time to Peak Elevations	Time to Return to Baseline
Myoglobin	1-4 h	6-7 h	18-24 h
CTnI	3-12 h	10-24 h	3-10 d
CTnT	3-12 h	12-48 h	5-14 d
CKMB	4-12 h	10-24 h	48-72 h
CKMBiso	2-6 h	12 h	38 h

CTnI, CTnT = troponins of cardiac myofibrils; CPK-MB, MM = tissue isoforms of creatine kinase.

C. **Unstable angina**. Patients with cardiac biomarker elevations and unstable angina are considered to have an NSTEMI and should be treated appropriately.

D. Treadmill stress testing and echocardiography is recommended for patients with a suspicion of coronary ischemia.

Heart Failure Caused by Systolic Left Ventricular Dysfunction

Over four million persons have HF in the United States. The mortality rate is 50 percent at two years and 60 to 70 percent at three years. Heart failure (HF) can result from any structural or functional cardiac disorder that impairs the ability of the ventricle to fill with or eject blood. It is characterized by dyspnea and fatigue, and signs of fluid retention.

I. Classification of severity

A. The classification system that is most commonly used to quantify the degree of functional limitation imposed by heart failure is the New York Heart Association (NYHA) classification.

Classification of Patients with Heart Failure Caused by Left Ventricular Dysfunction

New classification based on symptoms	Corresponding NYHA class
Asymptomatic	NYHA class I
Symptomatic	NYHA class II/III
Symptomatic with recent history of dyspnea at rest	NYHA class IIIb
Symptomatic with dyspnea at rest	NYHA class IV

B. Etiology. There are two mechanisms by which reduced cardiac output and heart failure occur: systolic dysfunction and diastolic dysfunction.

C. Systolic dysfunction. The most common causes of systolic dysfunction are coronary (ischemic) heart disease, idiopathic dilated cardiomyopathy, hypertension, and valvular disease. Coronary disease and hypertension account for 62 and 10 percent of cases, respectively.

D. Diastolic dysfunction can be induced by many of the same conditions that lead to systolic dysfunction. The most common causes are hypertension, ischemic heart disease, hypertrophic obstructive cardiomyopathy, and restrictive cardiomyopathy.

II. Clinical evaluation

A. There are two major classes of symptoms in HF: those due to excess fluid accumulation (dyspnea, edema, hepatic congestion, and ascites) and those due to a reduction in cardiac output (fatigue, weakness) that is most pronounced with exertion.

B. Acute and subacute presentations (days to weeks) are characterized primarily by shortness of breath, at rest and/or with exertion. Also common are orthopnea, paroxysmal nocturnal dyspnea, and, with right heart failure, right upper quadrant discomfort due to acute hepatic congestion, which can be confused with acute cholecystitis. Patients with atrial and/or ventricular tachyarrhythmias may complain of palpitations with or without lightheadedness.

C. Chronic presentations (months) differ in that fatigue, anorexia, bowel distension, and peripheral edema may be more pronounced than dyspnea.

D. Classic exertional angina usually indicates ischemic heart disease.

E. Acute heart failure after an antecedent flu-like illness suggests viral myocarditis.

F. Long-standing hypertension or alcohol use suggests hypertensive or alcoholic cardiomyopathy.

G. Amyloidosis should be excluded in patients who also have a history of heavy proteinuria.

H. Primary valvular dysfunction should be considered in a patient with significant murmurs.

I. Heart failure may be provoked or worsened by drugs, including antiarrhythmic agents such as disopyramide and flecainide; calcium channel blockers, particularly verapamil; beta-blockers; and nonsteroidal anti-inflammatory drugs (NSAIDs).

Factors Associated with Worsening Heart Failure
Cardiovascular factors
Superimposed ischemia or infarction Uncontrolled hypertension Unrecognized primary valvular disease Worsening secondary mitral regurgitation New onset or unctontrolled atrial fibrillation Excessive tachycardia Pulmonary embolism
Systemic factors
Inappropriate medications Superimposed infection Anemia Uncontrolled diabetes Thyroid dysfunction Electrolyte disorders Pregnancy
Patient-related factors
Medication noncompliance Dietary indiscretion Alcohol consumption Substance abuse

III. **Physical examination**

A. Patients compensate for a fall in cardiac output by increasing sympathetic outflow. This results in shunting of the cardiac output to vital organs, leading to sinus tachycardia, diaphoresis, and peripheral vasoconstriction, manifested as cool, pale, and sometimes cyanotic extremities.

B. **Volume overload.** There are three major manifestations of volume overload in patients with HF are pulmonary congestion, peripheral edema, and elevated jugular venous pressure.

C. **Ventricular enlargement.** Ventricular chamber size can be estimated by precordial palpation. An apical impulse that is laterally displaced past the midclavicular line is usually indicative of left ventricular enlargement. Left ventricular dysfunction can also lead to sustained apical impulse which may be accompanied by a parasternal heave.

D. **Pulmonary hypertension.** Patients with chronic heart failure often develop secondary pulmonary hypertension, which can contribute to dyspnea. These patients may also complain of substernal chest pressure, typical of angina. Physical signs of pulmonary hypertension can include increased intensity of P2, a murmur of pulmonary insufficiency, and a palpable pulmonic tap.

IV. Blood tests

A. Recommended initial blood tests for patients with signs or symptoms of HF include:

1. A complete blood count since anemia can exacerbate pre-existing HF.
2. Serum electrolytes and creatinine as a baseline to follow when initiating therapy with diuretics and/or angiotensin converting enzyme inhibitors.
3. Liver function tests, which may be affected by hepatic congestion.
4. Fasting blood glucose to detect underlying diabetes mellitus. (See "Heart failure in diabetes mellitus").

Laboratory Workup for Suspected Heart Failure

Blood urea nitrogen	Thyroid-stimulating hormone
Cardiac enzymes (CK-MB, troponin)	Urinalysis
Complete blood cell count	Echocardiogram
Creatinine	Electrocardiography
Electrolytes	Impedance cardiography
Liver function tests	Atrial natriuretic peptide (ANP)
Magnesium	Brain natriuretic peptide (BNP)

B. In addition, if it is determined that dilated cardiomyopathy is responsible for HF and the cause is not apparent, several other blood tests may be warranted.

1. Thyroid function tests, particularly in patients over the age of 65 or in patients with atrial fibrillation. Thyrotoxicosis is associated with atrial fibrillation and hypothyroidism may present as HF.
2. Iron studies (ferritin and TIBC) to screen for hereditary hemochromatosis (HH).

C. Other studies that may be undertaken depending upon the potential findings identified in the history and physical examination include:

1. ANA and other serologic tests for lupus.
2. Viral serologies and antimyosin antibody if myocarditis is suspected.
3. Evaluation for pheochromocytoma.
4. Thiamine, carnitine, and selenium levels.
5. Genetic testing and counseling (eg, in patients suspected of familial cardiomyopathy after obtaining a detailed family history).

D. **Plasma BNP.** With chronic HF, atrial myocytes secrete increased amounts of atrial natriuretic peptide (ANP) and ventricular myocytes secrete both ANP and brain natriuretic peptide (BNP) in response to the high atrial and ventricular filling pressures. The plasma concentrations of both hormones are increased in asymptomatic and symptomatic left ventricular dysfunction, permitting their use in diagnosis. A value BNP >100 pg/mL diagnoses HF with a sensitivity, specificity, and predictive accuracy of 90, 76, and 83 percent, respectively.

E. **Plasma N-pro-BNP.** The active BNP hormone is cleaved from the C-terminal end of its prohormone, pro-BNP. The N-terminal fragment, N-pro-BNP, is also released into the circulation. In normal subjects, the plasma concentrations of BNP and N-pro-BNP are similar (approximately 10 pmol/L). However, in patients with LV dysfunction, plasma N-pro-BNP concentrations are approximately four-fold higher than BNP concentrations.

V. Chest x-ray. The chest x-ray is a useful first diagnostic test, particularly in the evaluation of patients who present with dyspnea, to differentiate heart failure from primary pulmonary disease. Findings suggestive of heart failure include cardiomegaly (cardiac-to-thoracic width ratio above 50 percent), cephalization of the pulmonary vessels, Kerley B-lines, and pleural effusions. The cardiac size and silhouette may also reveal cardiomegaly.

VI. Electrocardiogram

A. The electrocardiogram may show findings that favor the presence of a specific cause of heart failure and can also detect arrhythmias such as asymptomatic ventricular premature beats, runs of nonsustained ventricular tachycardia, or atrial fibrillation, which may be the cause of or exacerbate HF.

B. Patients with dilated cardiomyopathy frequently have first degree AV block, left bundle branch block, left anterior fascicular block, or a nonspecific intraventricular conduction abnormality. Among the potentially diagnostic findings on ECG are:

1. Evidence of ischemic heart disease.
2. Left ventricular hypertrophy due to hypertension; a pseudo-infarct pattern may also be present.
3. Low-limb lead voltage on the surface ECG with a pseudo-infarction pattern (loss of precordial R-wave progression in leads V1-V6) can suggest an infiltrative process such as amyloidosis.
4. Low-limb lead voltage with precordial criteria for left ventricular hypertrophy is most suggestive of idiopathic dilated cardiomyopathy. A widened QRS complex and/or a left bundle branch block pattern is also consistent with this diagnosis.
5. Heart block, that may be complete, and various types of intraventricular conduction defects are observed in patients with cardiac sarcoidosis.
6. Persistent tachycardia such as atrial fibrillation with a rapid ventricular response may lead to a cardiomyopathy (tachycardia-mediated cardiomyopathy).

C. Most patients with HF due to systolic dysfunction have a significant abnormality on ECG. A normal ECG makes systolic dysfunction extremely unlikely (98 percent negative predictive value).

VII. Laboratory testing

A. **Echocardiography.** Echocardiography should be performed in all patients with new onset heart failure and can provide important information about ventricular size and function. The sensitivity and specificity echocardiography for the diagnosis of HF are as high as 80 and 100 percent, respectively.

B. **Detection of coronary heart disease.** Most patients with HF due to ischemic cardiomyopathy have known coronary heart disease. However, occult disease is a not uncommon cause of dilated cardiomyopathy, accounting for as many as 7 percent of initially unexplained cases. Heart failure resulting from coronary disease is usually irreversible due to myocardial infarction and subsequent ventricular remodeling. However, revascularization may be of benefit in patients in whom hibernating myocardium is in part responsible for the decline in myocardial function.

1. **Exercise testing** should be part of the initial evaluation of any patient with HF. In addition to detection of ischemic heart disease, assessment of exercise capacity can be used for risk stratification and determining prognosis. With severe heart failure, measurement of the maximal

oxygen uptake (VO$_2$max) provides an objective estimate of the functional severity of the myocardial dysfunction.

2. **Cardiac catheterization.** Coronary catheterization with angiography is indicated in virtually all patients with new onset heart failure of uncertain cause, even in patients with no history of anginal symptoms and a normal exercise test. Some exceptions include patients with comorbid conditions that either render catheterization too risky or that would preclude invasive therapy.

VIII. **Treatment of heart failure due to systolic dysfunction**

A. **Treatment of the underlying cardiac disease**

1. **Hypertension** is the primary cause of HF in 13 percent of patients.
2. Angiotensin converting enzyme (ACE) inhibitors, beta-blockers, and angiotensin II receptor blockers (ARBs) are the preferred antihypertensive agents because they improve survival in patients with HF. Beta-blockers can also provide anginal relief in patients with ischemic heart disease and rate control in atrial fibrillation. Beta-blocker therapy should always be initiated at very low doses.
3. **Renovascular disease testing** is indicated in patients in whom the history is suggestive (severe or refractory hypertension, a sudden rise in blood pressure, or repeated episodes of flash pulmonary edema).
4. **Ischemic heart disease.** Coronary atherosclerosis is the most common cause of cardiomyopathy, comprising 50 to 75 percent of patients with HF. All patients with ischemic heart disease should be treated medically for relief of angina and with risk-factor reduction. Myocardial revascularization with angioplasty or bypass surgery may improve symptom status, exercise capacity. Revascularization should also be considered in patients with a history of repeated episodes of acute left ventricular dysfunction and flash pulmonary edema.
5. **Valvular disease** is the primary cause of HF in 10 to 12 percent of patients. Surgical correction of valvular disease can lead to improvement in cardiac function.
6. **Other factors** that can cause, or worsen, HF include alcohol abuse, cocaine abuse, obstructive sleep apnea, nutritional deficiencies, myocarditis, hemochromatosis, sarcoidosis, and rheumatologic disorders, such as systemic lupus erythematosus.

Treatment Classification of Patients with Heart Failure Caused by Left Ventricular Systolic Dysfunction	
Symptoms	**Pharmacology**
Asymptomatic	ACE inhibitor or angiotensin-receptor blocker Beta blocker
Symptomatic	ACE inhibitor or angiotensin-receptor blocker Beta blocker Diuretic If symptoms persist: digoxin (Lanoxin)

Symptoms	Pharmacology
Symptomatic with recent history of dyspnea at rest	Diuretic ACE inhibitor or angiotensin-receptor blocker Spironolactone (Aldactone) Beta blocker Digoxin
Symptomatic with dyspnea at rest	Diuretic ACE inhibitor or angiotensin-receptor blocker Spironolactone (Aldactone) Digoxin

Dosages of Primary Drugs Used in the Treatment of Heart Failure

Drug	Starting Dosage	Target Dosage
Drugs that decrease mortality and improve symptoms		
ACE inhibitors		
Captopril (Capoten)	6.25 mg three times daily (one-half tablet)	12.5 to 50 mg three times daily
Enalapril (Vasotec)	2.5 mg twice daily	10 mg twice daily
Lisinopril (Zestril)	5 mg daily	10 to 20 mg daily
Ramipril (Altace)	1.25 mg twice daily	5 mg twice daily
Trandolapril (Mavik)	1 mg daily	4 mg daily
Angiotensin-Receptor Blockers (ARBs)		
Candesartan (Atacand)	4 mg bid	16 mg bid
Irbesartan (Avapro)	75 mg qd	300 mg qd
Losartan (Cozaar)	12.5 mg bid	50 mg bid
Valsartan (Diovan)	40 mg bid	160 mg bid
Telmisartan (Micardis)	20 mg qd	80 mg qd
Aldosterone antagonists		
Spironolactone (Aldactone)	25 mg daily	25 mg daily
Eplerenone (Inspra)	25 mg daily	25 mg daily
Beta blockers		
Bisoprolol (Zebeta)	1.25 mg daily (one-fourth tablet)	10 mg daily
Carvedilol (Coreg)	3.125 mg twice daily	25 to 50 mg twice daily
Metoprolol tartrate (Lopressor)	12.5 mg twice daily (one-fourth tablet)	50 to 75 mg twice daily
Metoprolol succinate (Toprol-XL)	12.5 mg daily (one-half tablet)	200 mg daily
Drugs that treat symptoms		
Thiazide diuretics		
Hydrochlorothiazide (Esidrex)	25 mg daily	25 to 100 mg daily

Drug	Starting Dosage	Target Dosage
Metolazone (Zaroxolyn)	2.5 mg daily	2.5 to 10 mg daily
Loop diuretics		
Bumetanide (Bumex)	1 mg daily	1 to 10 mg once to three times daily
Ethacrynic acid (Edecrin)	25 mg daily	25 to 200 mg once or twice daily
Furosemide (Lasix)	40mg daily	40 to 400 mg once to three times daily
Torsemide (Demadex)	20 mg daily	20 to 200 mg once or twice daily
Inotrope		
Digoxin (Lanoxin)	0.125 mg daily	0.125 to 0.375 mg daily

B. Pharmacologic therapy of heart failure

1. **ACE inhibitors** improve survival in patients with all severities of myocardial disease, ranging from asymptomatic left ventricular dysfunction to moderate or severe HF. All patients with asymptomatic or symptomatic left ventricular dysfunction should be started on an ACE inhibitor. Beginning therapy with low doses (eg, 2.5 mg of enalapril (Vasotec) BID or 6.25 mg of captopril (Capoten) TID) will reduce the likelihood of hypotension and azotemia. The dose is then gradually increased to a maintenance dose of 10 mg BID of enalapril, 50 mg TID of captopril, or up to 40 mg/day of lisinopril or quinapril.

2. **Angiotensin II receptor blockers** for the treatment of HF appear to be as effective as, or possibly slightly less effective than, ACE inhibitors. The addition of an ARB, if tolerated, to HF therapy in patients who are stable on ACE inhibitors and beta-blockers is recommended. ARB therapy should not be added to an ACE inhibitor in the immediate post-MI setting.

3. **Beta-blockers** carvedilol, metoprolol, and bisoprolol improve overall and event-free survival in patients with New York Heart Association (NYHA) class II to III HF and probably in class IV HF. Beta-blockers with intrinsic sympathomimetic activity (such as pindolol and acebutolol) should be avoided

   a. Carvedilol, metoprolol, or bisoprolol is recommended for all patients with symptomatic HF, unless contraindicated.

   b. Relative contraindications in HF include:
      (1) Heart rate <60 bpm.
      (2) Systolic arterial pressure <100 mm Hg.
      (3) Signs of peripheral hypoperfusion.
      (4) PR interval >0.24 sec.
      (5) Second- or third-degree atrioventricular block.
      (6) Severe chronic obstructive pulmonary disease.
      (7) History of asthma.
      (8) Severe peripheral vascular disease.

   c. Prior to initiation of therapy, the patient should be stable on an ACE inhibitor and (if necessary for symptom control) digoxin and diuretics, should have no or minimal evidence of fluid retention, and should not have required recent intravenous inotropic therapy.

    d. Therapy should be begun at very low doses and the dose doubled at regular intervals every two to three weeks until the target dose is reached or symptoms become limiting. Initial and target doses are:

        (1) Carvedilol (Coreg), 3.125 mg BID and 25 to 50 mg BID (the higher dose being used in subjects over 85 kg).

        (2) Metoprolol (Toprol), 6.25 mg BID and 50 to 75 mg BID, and for extended-release metoprolol, 12.5 or 25 mg daily and 200 mg/day.

        (3) Bisoprolol (Ziac), 1.25 mg QD and 5 to 10 mg QD.

        (4) The patient should weigh himself daily and call the physician if there has been a 1 to 1.5 kg weight gain. Weight gain may be treated with diuretics, but resistant edema or more severe decompensation may require dose reduction or cessation of the beta-blocker.

4. Digoxin is given to patients with HF and systolic dysfunction to control symptoms (fatigue, dyspnea, and exercise intolerance) and, in atrial fibrillation, to control the ventricular rate. Digoxin should be started in left ventricular systolic dysfunction (left ventricular ejection fraction [LVEF] <40 percent) who continue to have symptoms despite appropriate therapy including an ACE inhibitor, beta-blocker, and, if necessary for fluid control, a diuretic. The usual daily dose is 0.125 to 0.25 mg, based upon renal function. The serum digoxin concentration should be maintained between 0.5 and 0.8 ng/mL.

5. Diuretics. Sodium and water retention lead to pulmonary and peripheral edema.

    a. A loop diuretic should be given to control pulmonary and/or peripheral edema. The most commonly used loop diuretic is furosemide (Lasix), but some patients respond better to bumetanide (Bumex) or torsemide (Demadex) because of superior and more predictable absorption.

    b. The usual starting dose in outpatients with HF is 20 to 40 mg of furosemide. In patients who are volume overloaded, a reasonable goal is weight reduction of 0.5 to 1.0 kg/day. If a patient does not respond, the diuretic dose should initially be increased.

    c. In patients with HF and a normal glomerular filtration rate, the maximum doses are 40 to 80 mg of furosemide, 2 to 3 mg of bumetanide, or 20 to 50 mg of torsemide. In patients with renal insufficiency, a higher maximum dose of 160 to 200 mg of furosemide or its equivalent can be given.

    d. Intravenous diuretics (either as a bolus or a continuous infusion) are more potent than their equivalent oral doses and may be required for unstable or severe disease. Thiazide diuretics can be added for a synergistic effect.

    e. A continuous infusion of a loop diuretic may improve diuresis and reduce toxicity when compared to intermittent bolus injections. Urine output is significantly greater.

6. Aldosterone antagonists. Spironolactone and eplerenone, which compete with aldosterone for the mineralocorticoid receptor, prolong survival in selected patients with HF. Eplerenone has greater specificity for the mineralocorticoid receptor and a lower incidence of endocrine side effects.

    a. Therapy should be initiated with spironolactone, and switch to eplerenone (25 to 50 mg/day) if endocrine side effects occur. The serum potassium should be monitored.

C. Drugs that are contraindicated in HF

1. **Nonsteroidal anti-inflammatory drugs** (NSAIDs) can cause a worsening of pre-existing HF because of systemic vasoconstriction. NSAID may blunt the renal effects of diuretics and may reverse the effect of angiotensin converting enzyme (ACE) inhibitors.

2. **Thiazolidinediones** are oral hypoglycemic agents that increase insulin sensitivity. Drugs in this class cause fluid retention, which may precipitate HF. Patients with HF who are currently taking thiazolidinediones should be carefully followed for signs and symptoms of HF, and the agent should be stopped if signs of fluid retention develop. Thiazolidinediones should not be used in patients with New York Heart Association class III or IV HF.

3. **Metformin (Glucophage).** Patients with HF who take metformin are at increased risk of potentially lethal lactic acidosis. Metformin is contraindicated in patients with HF.

4. **Cilostazol** suppresses platelet aggregation and is a direct arterial vasodilator. In patients with HF, oral phosphodiesterase inhibitors has been associated with increased mortality. HF of any severity is a contraindication to the use of cilostazol.

5. **Sildenafil (Viagra)** is a phosphodiesterase inhibitor that is used in the treatment of impotence. The drug is a vasodilator that can lower systemic blood pressure. Sildenafil may be potentially hazardous in HF.

6. **Antiarrhythmic agents.** Most antiarrhythmic drugs have some negative inotropic activity and can precipitate HF. The further reduction in LV function can also impair the elimination of these drugs, resulting in drug toxicity. In addition, some antiarrhythmic drugs have a proarrhythmic effect. Amiodarone is safe and is the preferred drug to treat ventricular arrhythmias in HF

D. Lifestyle modification

1. Cessation of smoking.
2. Restriction of alcohol consumption.
3. Salt restriction to 2 to 3 g of sodium per day to minimize fluid accumulation.
4. Water restriction in patients who are hyponatremic may minimize pulmonary congestion.
5. Daily weight monitoring to detect fluid accumulation before it becomes symptomatic.
6. Weight reduction in obese subjects with a goal of being within 10 percent of ideal body weight.
7. A cardiac rehabilitation program for stable patients.

IX. Management of refractory HF

A. Intravenous inotropes and vasodilators. Patients with decompensated HF are often hospitalized and an intravenous infusion of a positive inotropic agent and/or a vasodilator is initiated. Inotropic drugs, such as dobutamine, dopamine, milrinone, and amrinone, and vasodilators, such as nitroprusside, nitroglycerin, and nesiritide, can acutely improve hemodynamics and relieve symptoms.

B. Symptomatic improvement has been demonstrated in patients after treatment with a continuous infusion of dobutamine (5 to 7.5 µg/kg per min) for three to five days. The benefit can last for 30 days or more. There is no evidence for a survival benefit, and intermittent, dobutamine may increase mortality. Use of intravenous dobutamine or milrinone is limited to the in-patient management of severe decompensated heart failure.

Treatment of Acute Heart Failure/Pulmonary Edema

- Oxygen therapy, 2 L/min by nasal canula
- Furosemide (Lasix) 20-80 mg IV
- Nitroglycerine start at 10-20 mcg/min and titrate to BP (use with caution if inferior/right ventricular infarction suspected)
- Sublingual nitroglycerin 0.4 mg
- Morphine sulfate 2-4 mg IV. Avoid if inferior wall MI suspected or if hypotensive or presence of tenuous airway
- Potassium supplementation prn

Atrial Fibrillation

Atrial fibrillation (AF) is more prevalent in men and with increasing age. AF can have adverse consequences related to a reduction in cardiac output and to atrial thrombus formation that can lead to systemic embolization.

I. Classification

A. Atrial fibrillation occurs in the normal heart and in the presence of organic heart disease. Classification of Atrial fibrillation:

1. **Paroxysmal (ie, self-terminating) AF** in which the episodes of AF generally last less than seven days (usually less than 24 hours) and may be recurrent.
2. **Persistent AF** fails to self-terminate and lasts for longer than seven days. Persistent AF may also be paroxysmal if it recurs after reversion. AF is considered recurrent when the patient experiences two or more episodes.
3. **Permanent AF** is considered to be present if the arrhythmia lasts for more than one year and cardioversion either has not been attempted or has failed.
4. **"Lone" AF** describes paroxysmal, persistent, or permanent AF in individuals without structural heart disease.

B. If the AF is secondary to cardiac surgery, pericarditis, myocardial infarction (MI), hyperthyroidism, pulmonary embolism, pulmonary disease, or other reversible causes, therapy is directed toward the underlying disease as well as the AF.

II. Clinical evaluation

A. History and physical examination. Associated symptoms with AF should be sought; the clinical type or "pattern" should be defined; the onset or date of discovery of the AF; the frequency and duration of AF episodes; any precipitating causes and modes of termination of AF; the response to drug therapy; and the presence of heart disease or potentially reversible causes (eg, hyperthyroidism).

B. The frequency and duration of AF episodes are determined from the history. Symptoms include palpitations, weakness, dizziness, and dyspnea. However, among patients with paroxysmal AF, up to 90% of episodes are not recognized by the patient.

C. **Electrocardiogram** is used to verify the presence of AF; identify left ventricular hypertrophy, pre-excitation, bundle branch block, or prior MI; define P-wave duration and morphology as well as other atrial arrhythmias on earlier ECGs.

D. **Chest x-ray** may be useful in assessing the lungs, vasculature, and cardiac outline.

E. **Echocardiogram.** The transthoracic echocardiography is required to evaluate the size of the right and left atria and the size and function of the right and left ventricles; to detect possible valvular heart disease, left ventricular hypertrophy, and pericardial disease; and to assess peak right ventricular pressure. It may also identify a left atrial thrombus, although the sensitivity is low. Transesophageal echocardiography is much more sensitive for atrial thrombi and can be used to determine the need for three to four weeks of anticoagulation prior to cardioversion.

F. **Assessment for hyperthyroidism.** A low-serum thyroid-stimulating hormone (TSH) value is found in 5.4% of patients with AF; only 1% have clinical hyperthyroidism. Measurement of serum TSH and free T4 is indicated in all patients with a first episode of AF, when the ventricular response to AF is difficult to control, or when AF recurs unexpectedly after cardioversion. Patients with low values (<0.5 mU/L) and normal serum free T4 probably have subclinical hyperthyroidism.

G. **Additional testing**
   1. Exercise testing is often used to assess the adequacy of rate control in permanent AF, to reproduce exercise-induced AF, and to evaluate for ischemic heart disease.
   2. Holter monitoring or event recorders are used to identify the arrhythmia if it is intermittent and not captured on routine electrocardiography.
   3. Electrophysiologic studies may be required with wide QRS complex tachycardia or a possible predisposing arrhythmia, such as atrial flutter or a paroxysmal supraventricular tachycardia.

III. **General treatment issues**

Risk-based Approach to Antithrombotic Therapy in Atrial Fibrillation	
Patient features	**Antithrombotic therapy**
Age <60 years No heart disease (line AF)	Aspirin (325 mg per day) or no therapy
Age <60 years Hear disease by no risk factors*	Aspirin (325 mg per day)
Age ≥60 years No risk factors*	Aspirin (325 mg per day)
Age ≥60 years With diabetes mellitus or CAD	Oral anticoagulation (INR 2 to 3) Addition of aspirin, 81 to 162 mg/day is optional
Age ≥75 years, especially women	Oral anticoagulation (INR ≈ 2.0)

Patient features	Antithrombotic therapy
Heart failure (HF) LVEF ≤0.35 Thyrotoxicosis Hypertension	Oral anticoagulation (INR 2 to 3)
Rheumatic heart disease (mitral stenosis) Prosthetic heart valves Prior thromboembolism Persistent atrial thrombus on TEE	Oral anticoagulation (INR 2.5 to 3.5 or higher may be apropriate)

*Risk factors for thromboembolism include heart failure, left ventricular ejection fraction (LVEF) less than 0.35, and hypertension.

A. Rate control with chronic anticoagulation is recommended for the majority of patients with AF.
B. Beta-blockers (eg, atenolol or metoprolol), diltiazem, and verapamil are recommended for rate control at both rest and exercise; digoxin is not effective during exercise and should be used in patients with heart failure or as a second-line agent.
C. Anticoagulation should be achieved with adjusted-dose warfarin unless the patient is considered at low embolic risk or has a contraindication. Aspirin may be used in such patients.
D. When rhythm control is chosen, both DC and pharmacologic cardioversion are appropriate options. To prevent dislodgment of pre-existing thrombi, warfarin therapy should be given for three to four weeks prior to cardioversion unless transesophageal echocardiography demonstrates no left atrial thrombi. Anticoagulation is continued for at least one month after cardioversion to prevent de novo thrombus formation.
E. After cardioversion, antiarrhythmic drugs to maintain sinus rhythm are not recommended, since the risks outweigh the benefits, except for patients with persistent symptoms during rate control that interfere with the patient's quality of life. Recommended drugs are amiodarone, disopyramide, propafenone, and sotalol.

IV. **Rhythm control**
A. **Reversion to NSR.** Patients with AF of more than 48 hours duration or unknown duration may have atrial thrombi that can embolize. In such patients, cardioversion should be delayed until the patient has been anticoagulated at appropriate levels for three to four weeks or transesophageal echocardiography has excluded atrial thrombi.
   1. DC cardioversion is indicated in patients who are hemodynamically unstable. In stable patients in whom spontaneous reversion due to correction of an underlying disease is not likely, either DC or pharmacologic cardioversion can be performed. Electrical cardioversion is usually preferred because of greater efficacy and a low risk of proarrhythmia. The overall success rate of electrical cardioversion for AF is 75 to 93 percent and is related inversely both to the duration of AF and to left atrial size.
   2. A number of antiarrhythmic drugs are more effective than placebo, converting 30 to 60 percent of patients. Evidence of efficacy is best

established for dofetilide, flecainide, ibutilide, propafenone, amiodarone, and quinidine.

3. Rate control with an atrioventricular (AV) nodal blocker (beta-blocker, diltiazem, or verapamil), or (if the patient has heart failure or hypotension) digoxin should be attained before instituting a class IA drug.

B. Maintenance of NSR. Only 20 to 30 percent of patients who are successfully cardioverted maintain NSR for more than one year without chronic antiarrhythmic therapy. This is more likely to occur in patients with AF for less than one year, no enlargement of the left atrium (ie, ≤ 4.0 cm), and a reversible cause of AF such as hyperthyroidism, pericarditis, pulmonary embolism, or cardiac surgery.

1. Prophylactic antiarrhythmic drug therapy is indicated only in patients who have a moderate-to-high risk for recurrence because the risks generally outweigh the benefits of maintenance antiarrhythmic drug therapy except in patients with persistent symptoms on a rate control regimen.

2. Evidence of efficacy is best for amiodarone, propafenone, disopyramide, sotalol, flecainide, and quinidine. Flecainide may be preferred in patients with no or minimal heart disease, while amiodarone is preferred in patients with a reduced left ventricular (LV) ejection fraction or heart failure and sotalol in patients with coronary heart disease. Concurrent administration of an AV nodal blocker is indicated in patients who have demonstrated a moderate-to-rapid ventricular response to AF.

3. Amiodarone is significantly more effective for maintenance of sinus rhythm than other antiarrhythmic drugs. Amiodarone should be used as first-line therapy in patients without heart failure.

V. Rate control in chronic AF. Rapid ventricular rate in patients with AF should be prevented because of hemodynamic instability and/or symptoms.

A. Rate control in AF is usually achieved by slowing AV nodal conduction with a beta-blocker, diltiazem, verapamil, or, in patients with heart failure or hypotension, digoxin. Amiodarone is also effective in patients who are not cardioverted to NSR.

B. Heart rate control include:

1. Rest heart rate ≤ 80 beats/min.
2. 24-hour Holter average ≤ 100 beats/min and no heart rate >110% of the age-predicted maximum.
3. Heart rate ≤ 110 beats/min in six minute walk.

C. Nonpharmacologic approaches. The medical approaches to either rate or rhythm control described above are not always effective.

1. **Rhythm control.** Alternative methods to maintain NSR in patients who are refractory to conventional therapy include surgery, radiofrequency catheter ablation, and pacemakers.

2. **Rate control.** Radio-frequency AV nodal-His bundle ablation with permanent pacemaker placement or AV nodal conduction modification are nonpharmacologic therapies for achieving rate control in patients who do not respond to pharmacologic therapy.

Intravenous Agents for Heart Rate Control in Atrial Fibrillation

Drug	Loading Dose	Onset	Maintenance Dose	Major Side Effects
Diltiazem	0.25 mg/kg IV over 2 min	2–7 min	5–15 mg per hour infusion	Hypotension, heart block, HF
Esmolol	0.5 mg/kg over 1 min	1 min	0.05–0.2 mg/kg/min	Hypotension, heart block, bradycardia, asthma, HF
Metoprolol	2.5–5 mg IV bolus over 2 min up to 3 doses	5 min	5 mg IV q6h	Hypotension, heart block, bradycardia, asthma, HF
Verapamil	0.075–0.15 mg/kg IV over 2 min	3–5 min	5-10 mg IV q6h	Hypotension, heart block, HF
Digoxin	0.25 mg IV q2h, up to 1.5 mg	2 h	0.125–0.25 mg daily	Digitalis toxicity, heart block, bradycardia

Oral Agents for Heart Rate Control

Drug	Loading Dose	Usual Maintenance Dose	Major Side Effects
Digoxin	0.25 mg PO q2h ; up to 1.5 mg	0.125–0.375 mg daily	Digitalis toxicity, heart block, bradycardia
Diltiazem Extended Release	NA	120–360 mg daily	Hypotension, heart block, HF
Metoprolol	NA	25–100 mg BID	Hypotension, heart block, bradycardia, asthma, HF
Propranolol Extended Release	NA	80–240 mg daily	Hypotension, heart block, bradycardia, asthma, HF
Verapamil Extended Release	NA	120–360 mg daily	Hypotension, heart block, HF, digoxin interaction

Drug	Loading Dose	Usual Maintenance Dose	Major Side Effects
Amiodarone	800 mg daily for 1 wk 600 mg daily for 1 wk 400 mg daily for 4–6 wk	200 mg daily	Pulmonary toxicity, skin discoloration, hypo or hyperthyroidism, corneal deposits, optic neuropathy, warfarin interaction, proarrhythmia (QT prolongation)

VI. Prevention of systemic embolization

A. Anticoagulation during restoration of NSR

1. **AF for more than 48 hours or unknown duration.** Outpatients without a contraindication to warfarin who have been in AF for more than 48 hours should receive three to four weeks of warfarin prior to and after cardioversion. This approach is also recommended for patients with AF who have valvular disease, evidence of left ventricular dysfunction, recent thromboembolism, or when AF is of unknown duration, as in an asymptomatic patient.

   a. The recommended target INR is 2.5 (range 2.0 to 3.0). The INR should be ≥ 2.0 in the weeks before cardioversion.

   b. An alternative approach that eliminates the need for prolonged anticoagulation prior to cardioversion is the use of transesophageal echocardiography-guided cardioversion.

   c. Thus, the long-term recommendations for patients who have been cardioverted to NSR but are at high risk for thromboembolism are similar to those in patients with chronic AF, even though the patients are in sinus rhythm.

2. **AF for less than 48 hours.** A different approach with respect to anticoagulation can be used in low-risk patients (no mitral valve disease, severe left ventricular dysfunction, or history of recent thromboembolism) in whom there is reasonable certainty that AF has been present for less than 48 hours. Such patients have a low risk of clinical thromboembolism if converted early (0.8%), even without screening TEE.

3. Long-term anticoagulation prior to cardioversion is not recommended in such patients, but heparin use is recommended at presentation and during the pericardioversion period.

Antithrombotic Therapy in Cardioversion for Atrial Fibrillation	
Timing of cardioversion	**Anticoagulation**
Early cardioversion in patients with atrial fibrillation for less than 48 hours	Heparin during cardioversion period to achieve PTT of 50-70 seconds. Heparin 70 U/kg load, 15 U/kg/hr drip.
Early cardioversion in patients with atrial fibrillation for more than 48 hours or an unknown duration, but with documented absence of atrial thrombi	Heparin during cardioversion period to achieve PTT of 50-70 seconds. Warfarin (Coumadin) for 4 weeks after cardioversion to achieve target INR of 2.0 to 3.0.

Timing of cardioversion	Anticoagulation
Elective cardioversion in patients with atrial fibrillation for more than 48 hours or an unknown duration	Warfarin for 3 weeks before and 4 weeks after cardioversion to achieve target INR of of 2.0 to 3.0.

Weight-based nomogram for intravenous heparin infusion	
Initial dose	80 U/kg bolus, then 18 U/kg per hour
aPTT* <35 sec (<1.2 x control)	80 U/kg bolus, then increase infusion rate by 4 U/kg per hour
aPTT	40 U/kg per hour, then increase infusion by 2 U/kg per hour
aPTT	No change
aPTT	Decrease infusion rate by 2q U/kg per hour
aPTT	Hold infusion 1 hour, then decrease infusion rate by 3 U/kg per hour
*aPTT = activated partial thromboplastin time	

4. Current practice is to administer aspirin for a first episode of AF that converts spontaneously and warfarin for at least four weeks to all other patients.
5. Aspirin should not be considered in patients with AF of less than 48 hours duration if there is associated rheumatic mitral valve disease, severe left ventricular dysfunction, or recent thromboembolism. Such patients should be treated the same as patients with AF of longer duration: one month of oral anticoagulation with warfarin or shorter-term anticoagulation with screening TEE prior to elective electrical or pharmacologic cardioversion followed by prolonged warfarin therapy after cardioversion.

B. Anticoagulation in chronic AF

1. The incidence of stroke associated with AF is 3 to 5 percent per year in the absence of anticoagulation; compared with the general population, AF significantly increases the risk of stroke (relative risk 2.4 in men and 3.0 in women).
2. The incidence of stroke is relatively low in patients with AF who are under age 65 and have no risk factors. The prevalence of stroke associated with AF increases strikingly with age and with other risk factors including diabetes, hypertension, previous stroke as clinical risk factors, and left ventricular dysfunction. The risk appears to be equivalent in chronic and paroxysmal AF.
3. Choice of antiembolism therapy.
   a. Patients with a CHADS2 score of 0 are at low risk of embolization (0.5% per year) and can be managed with aspirin.

    b. Patients with a CHADS2 score >3 are at high risk (5.3 to 6.9 percent per year) and should, in the absence of a contraindication, be treated with warfarin.

    c. Patients with a CHADS2 score of 1 or 2 are at intermediate risk of embolization (1.5 to 2.5 percent per year). In this group, the choice between warfarin therapy and aspirin will depend upon many factors, including patient preference.

   4. An INR between 2.0 and 3.0 is recommended for most patients with AF who receive warfarin therapy. A higher goal (INR between 2.5 and 3.5) is reasonable for patients at particularly high risk for embolization (eg, prior thromboembolism, rheumatic heart disease, prosthetic heart valves). An exception to the latter recommendation occurs in patients over the age of 75 who are at increased risk for major bleeding. A target INR of 1.8 to 2.5 is recommended for this age group.

  C. Anticoagulation in paroxysmal AF. The stroke risk appears to be equivalent in paroxysmal and chronic AF. The factors governing the choice between warfarin and aspirin therapy and the intensity of warfarin therapy are similar to patients with chronic AF. Among patients with very infrequent and short episodes of AF, any protective effect from anticoagulation may be more than offset by bleeding risk.

VII. Presentation and management of recent onset AF

  A. Most patients with recent onset AF present with palpitations, a sense of the heart racing, fatigue, lightheadedness, increased urination, or mild shortness of breath. More severe symptoms and signs include dyspnea, angina, hypotension, presyncope, or infrequently syncope. In addition, some patients present with an embolic event or the insidious onset of right-sided heart failure (peripheral edema, weight gain, and ascites).

  B. Indications for hospitalization

   1. For the treatment of an associated medical problem, which is often the reason for the arrhythmia.

   2. For elderly patients who are more safely treated for AF in hospital.

   3. For patients with underlying heart disease who have hemodynamic consequences from the AF or who are at risk for a complication resulting from therapy of the arrhythmia.

  C. Search for an underlying cause, such as heart failure (HF), pulmonary problems, hypertension, or hyperthyroidism, and for the urgency for heart rate slowing.

  D. Serum should be obtained for measurement of thyroid stimulating hormone (TSH) and free T4. This should be done even if there are no symptoms suggestive of hyperthyroidism, since the risk of AF is increased up to threefold in patients with subclinical hyperthyroidism. The latter disorder is characterized by low serum TSH (<0.5 mU/L) and normal serum free T4.

  E. If AF appears to have been precipitated by a reversible medical problem, cardioversion should be postponed until the condition has been successfully treated, which will often lead to spontaneous reversion. If this treatment is to be initiated as an outpatient, anticoagulation with warfarin should be begun with cardioversion performed, if necessary, after three to four weeks of adequate anticoagulation. If the patient is to be admitted to the hospital for treatment of the underlying disease, it is prudent to begin heparin therapy and then institute oral warfarin. Cardioversion is again performed after three to four weeks of adequate anticoagulation if the patient does not revert to NSR. In either case, three to four weeks of adequate anticoagulation are not necessary if TEE is performed and shows no left atrial thrombus.

F. Indications for urgent cardioversion
   1. Active ischemia.
   2. Significant hypotension, to which poor LV systolic function, diastolic dysfunction, or associated mitral or aortic valve disease may contribute.
   3. Severe manifestations of HF.
   4. The presence of a pre-excitation syndrome, which may lead to an extremely rapid ventricular rate.
   5. In a patient who has truly urgent indications for cardioversion, the need for restoration of NSR takes precedence over the need for protection from thromboembolic risk. If feasible, the patient should still be heparinized for the cardioversion procedure.

G. Initial rate control with mild-to-moderate symptoms. Most patients with acute AF do not require immediate reversion. Initial treatment directed at slowing the ventricular rate will usually result in improvement of the associated symptoms. This can be achieved with beta-blockers, calcium channel blockers (verapamil and diltiazem), or digoxin. The drug selected and the route of administration (oral versus intravenous) are dictated by the clinical presentation.
   1. Digoxin is the preferred drug only in patients with AF due to HF. Digoxin can also be used in patients who cannot take or who respond inadequately to beta-blockers or calcium channel blockers. The effect of digoxin is additive to both these drugs.
   2. A beta-blocker, diltiazem, or verapamil is the preferred drug in the absence of HF. Beta-blockers are particularly useful when the ventricular response increases to inappropriately high rates during exercise, after an acute MI, and when exercise-induced angina pectoris is also present. A calcium channel blocker is preferred in patients with chronic lung disease. The use of both a beta-blocker and calcium channel blocker should be avoided.

H. Elective cardioversion. In some patients, antiarrhythmic drugs are administered prior to cardioversion to increase the chance of successful reversion and to prevent recurrence. Patients who are successfully cardioverted generally require antiarrhythmic drugs to increase the likelihood of maintaining sinus rhythm.

I. Immediate cardioversion. There is a low risk of systemic embolization if the duration of the arrhythmia is 48 hours or less and there are no associated cardiac abnormalities (mitral valve disease or LV enlargement). In such patients, electrical or pharmacologic cardioversion can be attempted after systemic heparinization. Aspirin should be administered for a first episode of AF that converts spontaneously and warfarin for at least four weeks to all other patients.

J. Delayed cardioversion. It is preferable to anticoagulate with warfarin for three to four weeks before attempted cardioversion to allow any left atrial thrombi to resolve if:
   1. The duration of AF is more than 48 hours or of unknown duration.
   2. There is associated mitral valve disease or significant cardiomyopathy or HF.
   3. The patient has a prior history of a thromboembolic event.
   4. During this time, rate control should be maintained with an oral AV nodal blocker. The recommended target INR is 2.5 (range 2.0 to 3.0). The INR should be consistently ≥ 2.0 in the weeks before cardioversion.

K. Role of TEE. TEE immediately prior to elective cardioversion should be considered for those patients at increased risk for left atrial thrombi (eg, rheumatic mitral valve disease, recent thromboembolism, severe LV systolic dysfunction). Among patients with AF of recent onset (but more than 48 hours) who are not being anticoagulated, an alternative approach to three to four weeks of warfarin therapy before cardioversion is TEE-based screening with cardioversion performed if no thrombi are seen.

Hypertensive Crisis

Severe hypertension is defined as an elevation in diastolic blood pressure (BP) higher than 130 mm Hg.

I. Clinical evaluation of severe hypertension

A. Hypertensive emergencies is defined by a diastolic blood pressure >120 mm Hg associated with ongoing vascular damage. Symptoms or signs of neurologic, cardiac, renal, or retinal dysfunction are present. Adequate blood pressure reduction is required within a few hours. Hypertensive emergencies include severe hypertension in the following settings:

1. Aortic dissection
2. Acute left ventricular failure and pulmonary edema
3. Acute renal failure or worsening of chronic renal failure
4. Hypertensive encephalopathy
5. Focal neurologic damage indicating thrombotic or hemorrhagic stroke
6. Pheochromocytoma, cocaine overdose, or other hyperadrenergic states
7. Unstable angina or myocardial infarction
8. Eclampsia

B. Hypertensive urgency is defined as diastolic blood pressure >130 mm Hg without evidence of vascular damage; the disorder is asymptomatic and no retinal lesions are present.

C. Secondary hypertension includes renovascular hypertension, pheochromocytoma, cocaine use, withdrawal from alpha-2 stimulants, clonidine, beta-blockers or alcohol, and noncompliance with antihypertensive medications.

II. Initial assessment of severe hypertension

A. When severe hypertension is noted, the measurement should be repeated in both arms to detect any significant differences. Peripheral pulses should be assessed for absence or delay, which suggests dissecting aortic dissection. Evidence of pulmonary edema should be sought.

B. Target organ damage is suggested by chest pain, neurologic signs, altered mental status, profound headache, dyspnea, abdominal pain, hematuria, focal neurologic signs (paralysis or paresthesia), or hypertensive retinopathy.

C. Prescription drug use should be assessed, including missed doses of antihypertensives. History of recent cocaine or amphetamine use should be sought.

D. If focal neurologic signs are present, a CT scan may be required to differentiate hypertensive encephalopathy from a stroke syndrome.

III. Laboratory evaluation

A. Complete blood cell count, urinalysis for protein, glucose, and blood; urine sediment examination; chemistry panel (SMA-18).

B. If chest pain is present, cardiac enzymes are obtained.

    C. If the history suggests a hyperadrenergic state, the possibility of a pheochromocytoma should be excluded with a 24-hour urine for catecholamines. A urine drug screen may be necessary to exclude illicit drug use.

    D. Electrocardiogram should be completed.

    E. Suspected primary aldosteronism can be excluded with a 24-hour urine potassium and an assessment of plasma renin activity. Renal artery stenosis can be excluded with captopril renography and intravenous pyelography.

IV. Management of hypertensive emergencies

    A. The patient should be hospitalized for intravenous access, continuous intra-arterial blood pressure monitoring, and electrocardiographic monitoring. Volume status and urinary output should be monitored. Rapid, uncontrolled reductions in blood pressure should be avoided because coma, stroke, myocardial infarction, acute renal failure, or death may result.

    B. The goal of initial therapy is to terminate ongoing target organ damage. The mean arterial pressure should be lowered not more than 20-25%, or to a diastolic blood pressure of 100 mm Hg over 15 to 30 minutes. Blood pressure should be controlled over a few hours.

V. Management of hypertensive urgencies

    A. The initial goal in patients with severe asymptomatic hypertension should be a reduction in blood pressure to 160/110 over several hours with conventional oral therapy.

    B. If the patient is not volume depleted, furosemide (Lasix) is given in a dosage of 20 mg if renal function is normal, and higher if renal insufficiency is present. A calcium channel blocker (isradipine ([DynaCirc], 5 mg or felodipine [Plendil], 5 mg) should be added. A dose of captopril (Capoten)(12.5 mg) can be added if the response is not adequate. This regimen should lower the blood pressure to a safe level over three to six hours and the patient can be discharged on a regimen of once-a-day medications.

VI. Parenteral antihypertensive agents

    A. Nitroprusside (Nipride)

       1. Nitroprusside is the drug of choice in almost all hypertensive emergencies (except myocardial ischemia or renal impairment). It dilates both arteries and veins, and it reduces afterload and preload. Onset of action is nearly instantaneous, and the effects disappear 1-2 minutes after discontinuation.

       2. The starting dosage is 0.25-0.5 mcg/kg/min by continuous infusion with a range of 0.25-8.0 mcg/kg/min. Titrate dose to gradually reduce blood pressure over minutes to hours.

       3. When treatment is prolonged or when renal insufficiency is present, the risk of cyanide and thiocyanate toxicity is increased. Signs of thiocyanate toxicity include disorientation, fatigue, hallucinations, nausea, toxic psychosis, and seizures.

    B. Nitroglycerin

       1. Nitroglycerin is the drug of choice for hypertensive emergencies with coronary ischemia. It should not be used with hypertensive encephalopathy because it increases intracranial pressure.

       2. Nitroglycerin increases venous capacitance, decreases venous return and left ventricular filling pressure. It has a rapid onset of action of 2-5 minutes. Tolerance may occur within 24-48 hours.

   3. The starting dose is 15 mcg IV bolus, then 5-10 mcg/min (50 mg in 250 mL D5W). Titrate by increasing the dose at 3- to 5-minute intervals. Generally doses $\geq$1.0 mcg/kg/min are required for afterload reduction (max 2.0 mcg/kg/hr). Monitor for methemoglobinemia.

C. Labetalol IV (Normodyne)
   1. Labetalol is a good choice if BP elevation is associated with hyperadrenergic activity, aortic dissection, an aneurysm, or post-operative hypertension.
   2. Labetalol is administered as 20 mg slow IV over 2 min. Additional doses of 20-80 mg may be administered q5-10min, then q3-4h prn or 0.5-2.0 mg/min IV infusion. Labetalol is contraindicated in obstructive pulmonary disease, CHF, or heart block greater than first degree.

D. Enalaprilat IV (Vasotec)
   1. Enalaprilat is an ACE-inhibitor with a rapid onset of action (15 min) and long duration of action (11 hours). It is ideal for patients with heart failure or accelerated-malignant hypertension.
   2. Initial dose, 1.25 mg IVP (over 2-5 min) q6h, then increase up to 5 mg q6h. Reduce dose in azotemic patients. Contraindicated in bilateral renal artery stenosis.

E. Esmolol (Brevibloc) is a non-selective beta-blocker with a 1-2 min onset of action and short duration of 10 min. The dose is 500 mcg/kg/min x 1 min, then 50 mcg/kg/min; max 300 mcg/kg/min IV infusion.

F. Hydralazine is a preload and afterload reducing agent. It is ideal in hypertension due to eclampsia. Reflex tachycardia is common. The dose is 20 mg IV/IM q4-6h.

G. Nicardipine (Cardene IV) is a calcium channel blocker. It is contraindicated in presence of CHF. Tachycardia and headache are common. The onset of action is 10 min, and the duration is 2-4 hours. The dose is 5 mg/hr continuous infusion, up to 15 mg/hr.

H. Fenoldopam (Corlopam) is a vasodilator. It may cause reflex tachycardia and headaches. The onset of action is 2-3 min, and the duration is 30 min. The dose is 0.01 mcg/kg/min IV infusion titrated, up to 0.3 mcg/kg/min.

I. Phentolamine (Regitine) is an intravenous alpha-adrenergic antagonist used in excess catecholamine states, such as pheochromocytomas, rebound hypertension due to withdrawal of clonidine, and drug ingestions. The dose is 2-5 mg IV every 5 to 10 minutes.

J. Trimethaphan (Arfonad) is a ganglionic-blocking agent. It is useful in dissecting aortic aneurysm when beta-blockers are contraindicated; however, it is rarely used because most physicians are more familiar with nitroprusside. The dosage of trimethoprim is 0.3-3 mg/min IV infusion.

Acute Pericarditis

Pericarditis is the most common disease of the pericardium. The most common cause of pericarditis is viral infection. This disorder is characterized by chest pain, a pericardial friction rub, electrocardiographic changes, and pericardial effusion.

I. Clinical features
  A. Chest pain of acute infectious (viral) pericarditis typically develops in younger adults 1 to 2 weeks after a "viral illness." The chest pain is of sudden and severe onset, with retrosternal and/or left precordial pain and referral to the back and trapezius ridge. Pain may be preceded by low-grade fever. Radiation to the arms may also occur. The pain is often pleuritic (eg, accentuated by inspiration or coughing) and may also be relieved by changes in posture (upright posture).
  B. A pericardial friction rub is the most important physical sign. It is often described as triphasic, with systolic and both early (passive ventricular filling) and late (atrial systole) diastolic components, or more commonly a biphasic (systole and diastole).
  C. Resting tachycardia (rarely atrial fibrillation) and a low-grade fever may be present.

Causes of Pericarditis	
Idiopathic	Hypersensitivity: drug
Infectious: Viral, bacterial, tubercu-	Postmyocardial injury syndrome
lous, parasitic, fungal	Trauma
Connective tissue diseases Meta-	Dissecting aneurysm
bolic: uremia, hypothyroidism Neo-	Chylopericardium
plasm, radiation	

II. Diagnostic testing
  A. **ECG changes.** During the initial few days, diffuse (limb leads and precordial leads) ST segment elevations are common in the absence of reciprocal ST segment depression. PR segment depression is also common and reflects atrial involvement.
  B. The chest radiograph is often unrevealing, although a small left pleural effusion may be seen. An elevated erythrocyte sedimentation rate and C-reactive protein (CRP) and mild elevations of the white blood cell count are also common.
  C. **Labs:** CBC, SMA 12, albumin, viral serologies: Coxsackie A & B, measles, mumps, influenza, ASO titer, hepatitis surface antigen, ANA, rheumatoid factor, anti-myocardial antibody, PPD with candida, mumps. Cardiac enzymes q8h x 4, ESR, blood C&S X 2.
  D. **Pericardiocentesis:** Gram stain, C&S, cell count & differential, cytology, glucose, protein, LDH, amylase, triglyceride, AFB, specific gravity, pH.
  E. **Echocardiography** is the most sensitive test for detecting pericardial effusion, which may occur with pericarditis.

III. Treatment of acute pericarditis (nonpurulent)
  A. If effusion present on echocardiography, pericardiocentesis should be performed and the catheter should be left in place for drainage.

B. Treatment of pain starts with nonsteroidal anti-inflammatory drugs, meperidine, or morphine. In some instances, corticosteroids may be required to suppress inflammation and pain.

C. Anti-inflammatory treatment with NSAIDs is first-line therapy.
   1. Indomethacin (Indocin) 25 mg tid or 75 mg SR qd, **OR**
   2. Ketorolac (Toradol) 15-30 mg IV q6h, **OR**
   3. Ibuprofen (Motrin) 600 mg q8h.

D. Morphine sulfate 5-15 mg intramuscularly every 4-6 hours. Meperidine (Demerol) may also be used, 50-100 mg IM/IV q4-6h prn pain and promethazine (Phenergan) 25-75 mg IV q4h.

E. Prednisone, 60 mg daily, to be reduced every few days to 40, 20, 10, and 5 mg daily.

F. Purulent pericarditis
   1. Nafcillin or oxacillin 2 gm IV q4h **AND EITHER**
   2. Gentamicin or tobramycin 100-120 mg IV (1.5-2 mg/kg); then 80 mg (1.0-1.5 mg/kg) IV q8h (adjust in renal failure) **OR**
   3. Ceftizoxime (Cefizox) 1-2 gm IV q8h.
   4. Vancomycin, 1 gm IV q12h, may be used in place of nafcillin or oxacillin.

Pacemakers

Indications for implantation of a permanent pacemaker are based on symptoms, the presence of heart disease and the presence of symptomatic bradyarrhythmias. Pacemakers are categorized by a three- to five-letter code according to the site of the pacing electrode and the mode of pacing.

I. Indications for pacemakers
   A. First-degree atrioventricular (AV) block can be associated with severe symptoms. Pacing may benefit patients with a PR interval greater than 0.3 seconds. Type I second-degree AV block does not usually require permanent pacing because progression to a higher degree AV block is not common. Permanent pacing improves survival in patients with complete heart block.
   B. Permanent pacing is not needed in reversible causes of AV block, such as electrolyte disturbances or Lyme disease. Implantation is easier and of lower cost with single-chamber ventricular demand (VVI) pacemakers, but use of these devices is becoming less common with the advent of dual-chamber demand (DDD) pacemakers.

Generic Pacemaker Codes				
Position 1 (chamber paced)	Position 2 (chamber sensed)	Position 3 (response to sensing)	Position 4 (programmable functions; rate modulation)	Position 5 (antitachyarrhythmia functions)
V--ventricle	V--ventricle	T--triggered	P--programmable rate and/or output	P--pacing (antitachyarrhythmia)
A--atrium	A--atrium	I--inhibited	M--multiprogrammability of rate, output, sensitivity, etc.	S--shock
D--dual (A & V)	D--dual (A & V)	D--dual (T & I)	C--communicating (telemetry)	D--dual (P + S)
O--none	O--none	O--none	R--rate modulation O--none	O--none

C. Sick sinus syndrome (or sinus node dysfunction) is the most common reason for permanent pacing. Symptoms are related to the bradyarrhythmias of sick sinus syndrome. VVI mode is typically used in patients with sick sinus syndrome, but recent studies have shown that DDD pacing improves morbidity, mortality and quality of life.

II. **Temporary pacemakers**
   A. Temporary pacemaker leads generally are inserted percutaneously, then positioned in the right ventricular apex and attached to an external generator. Temporary pacing is used to stabilize patients awaiting permanent pacemaker implantation, to correct a transient symptomatic bradycardia due to drug toxicity or to suppress Torsades de Pointes by maintaining a rate of 85-100 beats per minute until the cause has been eliminated.
   B. Temporary pacing may also be used in a prophylactic fashion in patients at risk of symptomatic bradycardia during a surgical procedure or high-degree AV block in the setting of an acute myocardial infarction.
   C. In emergent situations, ventricular pacing can be instituted immediately by transcutaneous pacing using electrode pads applied to the chest wall.

References: See page 168.

Pulmonary Disorders

T. Scott Gallacher, MD
Ryan Klein, MD
Michael Krutzik, MD
Thomas Vovan, MD

Orotracheal Intubation

Endotracheal Tube Size (interior diameter):
>   Women 7.0-9.0 mm
>   Men 8.0-10.0 mm

1. Prepare suction apparatus. Have Ambu bag and mask apparatus setup with 100% oxygen; and ensure that patient can be adequately bag ventilated and suction apparatus is available.
2. If sedation and/or paralysis is required, consider rapid sequence induction as follows:
   - **A.** Fentanyl (Sublimaze) 50 mcg increments IV (1 mcg/kg) with:
   - **B.** Midazolam (Versed) 1 mg IV q2-3 min. max 0.1-0.15 mg/kg followed by:
   - **C.** Succinylcholine (Anectine) 0.6-1.0 mg/kg, at appropriate intervals; or vecuronium (Norcuron) 0.1 mg/kg IV x 1.
   - **D.** Propofol (Diprivan): 0.5 mg/kg IV bolus.
   - **E.** Etomidate (Amidate): 0.3-0.4 mg/kg IV.
3. Position the patient's head in the sniffing position with head flexed at neck and extended. If necessary, elevate the head with a small pillow.
4. Ventilate the patient with bag mask apparatus and hyperoxygenate with 100% oxygen.
5. Hold laryngoscope handle with left hand, and use right hand to open the patient's mouth. Insert blade along the right side of mouth to the base of tongue, and push the tongue to the left. If using curved blade, advance it to the vallecula (superior to epiglottis), and lift anteriorly, being careful not to exert pressure on the teeth. If using a straight blade, place beneath the epiglottis and lift anteriorly.
6. Place endotracheal tube (ETT) into right corner of mouth and pass it through the vocal cords; stop just after the cuff disappears behind vocal cords. If unsuccessful after 30 seconds, stop and resume bag and mask ventilation before re-attempting. A stilette to maintain the shape of the ETT in a hockey stick shape may be used. Remove stilette after intubation.
7. Inflate cuff with syringe keeping cuff pressure <20 cm H_2O, and attach the tube to an Ambu bag or ventilator. Confirm bilateral, equal expansion of the chest and equal bilateral breath sounds. Auscultate the abdomen to confirm that the ETT is not in the esophagus. If there is any question about proper ETT location, repeat laryngoscopy with tube in place to be sure it is endotracheal. Remove the tube immediately if there is any doubt about proper location. Secure the tube with tape and note centimeter mark at the mouth. Suction the oropharynx and trachea.
8. Confirm proper tube placement with a chest x-ray (tip of ETT should be between the carina and thoracic inlet, or level with the top of the aortic notch).

Nasotracheal Intubation

Nasotracheal intubation is the preferred method of intubation if prolonged intubation is anticipated (increased patient comfort). Intubation will be facilitated if the patient is awake and spontaneously breathing. There is an increased incidence of sinusitis with nasotracheal intubation.

1. Spray the nasal passage with a vasoconstrictor such as cocaine 4% or phenylephrine 0.25% (Neo-Synephrine). If sedation is required before nasotracheal intubation, administer midazolam (Versed) 0.05-0.1 mg/kg IV push. Lubricate the nasal airway with lidocaine ointment.
   Tube Size:
   Women 7.0 mm tube
   Men 8.0, 9.0 mm tube
2. Place the nasotracheal tube into the nasal passage, and guide it into nasopharynx along a U-shaped path. Monitor breath sounds by listening and feeling the end of tube. As the tube enters the oropharynx, gradually guide the tube downward. If the breath sounds stop, withdraw the tube 1-2 cm until breath sounds are heard again. Reposition the tube, and, if necessary, extend the head and advance. If difficulty is encountered, perform direct laryngoscopy and insert tube under direct visualization.
3. Successful intubation occurs when the tube passes through the cords; a cough may occur and breath sounds will reach maximum intensity if the tube is correctly positioned. Confirm correct placement by checking for bilateral breath sounds and expansion of the chest.
4. Confirm proper tube placement with chest x-ray.

Respiratory Failure and Ventilator Management

I. **Indications for ventilatory support**. Respirations >35, vital capacity <15 mL/kg, negative inspiratory force <-25, pO_2 <60 on 50% O_2. pH <7.2, pCO_2 >55, severe, progressive, symptomatic hypercapnia and/or hypoxia, severe metabolic acidosis.

II. **Initiation of ventilator support**
   A. **Noninvasive positive pressure ventilation** may be safely utilized in acute hypercapnic respiratory failure, avoiding the need for invasive ventilation and accompanying complications. It is not useful in normocapnic or hypoxemic respiratory failure.
   B. **Intubation**
      1. **Prepare suction apparatus**, laryngoscope, endotracheal tube (No. 8); clear airway and place oral airway, hyperventilate with bag and mask attached to high-flow oxygen.
      2. **Midazolam (Versed)** 1-2 mg IV boluses until sedated.
      3. **Intubate**, inflate cuff, ventilate with bag, auscultate chest, and suction trachea.
   C. **Initial orders**
      1. **Assist control (AC)** 8-14 breaths/min, tidal volume = 750 mL (6 cc/kg ideal body weight), FiO_2 = 100%, PEEP = 3-5 cm H_2O, Set rate so that minute ventilation (VE) is approximately 10 L/min. Alternatively, use intermittent mandatory ventilation (IMV) mode with same tidal volume

and rate to achieve near-total ventilatory support. Pressure support at 5-15 cm H_2O in addition to IMV may be added.

2. **ABG** should be obtained. Check ABG for adequate ventilation and oxygenation. If PO_2 is adequate and pulse oximetry is >98%, then titrate FIO_2 to a safe level (FIO_2<60%) by observing the saturation via pulse oximetry. Repeat ABG when target FIO_2 is reached.

3. **Chest x-ray for tube placement**, measure cuff pressure q8h (maintain <20 mm Hg), pulse oximeter, arterial line, and/or monitor end tidal CO_2. Maintain oxygen saturation >90-95%.

Ventilator Management

A. **Decreased minute ventilation.** Evaluate patient and rule out complications (endotracheal tube malposition, cuff leak, excessive secretions, bronchospasms, pneumothorax, worsening pulmonary disease, sedative drugs, pulmonary infection). Readjust ventilator rate to maintain mechanically assisted minute ventilation of 10 L/min. If peak airway pressure (AWP) is >45 cm H_2O, decrease tidal volume to 7-8 L/kg (with increase in rate if necessary), or decrease ventilator flow rate.

B. **Arterial saturation >94% and pO_2 >100,** reduce FIO_2 (each 1% decrease in FIO_2 reduces pO_2 by 7 mm Hg); once FIO_2 is <60%, PEEP may be reduced by increments of 2 cm H_2O until PEEP is 3-5cm H_2O. Maintain O_2 saturation of >90% (pO_2 >60).

C. **Arterial saturation <90% and pO_2 <60,** increase FIO_2 up to 60-100%, then consider increasing PEEP by increments of 3-5 cm H_2O (PEEP >10 requires a PA catheter). Add additional PEEP until oxygenation is adequate with an FIO_2 of <60%.

D. **Excessively low pH,** (pH <7.33 because of respiratory acidosis/hypercapnia): Increase rate and/or tidal volume. Keep peak airway pressure <40-50 cm H_2O if possible.

E. **Excessively high pH** (>7.48 because of respiratory alkalosis/hypocapnia): Reduce rate and/or tidal volume. If the patient is breathing rapidly above ventilator rate, consider sedation.

F. **Patient "fighting ventilator":** Consider IMV or SIMV mode, or add sedation with or without paralysis. Paralytic agents should not be used without concurrent amnesia and/or sedation.

G. **Sedation**

   1. **Midazolam (Versed)** 0.05 mg/kg IVP x1, then 0.02-0.1 mg/kg/hr IV infusion. Titrate in increments of 25-50%.

   2. **Lorazepam (Ativan)** 1-2 mg IV ql-2h pm sedation or 0.05 mg/kg IVP x1, then 0.025-0.2 mg/kg/hr IV infusion. Titrate in increments of 25-50%.

   3. **Morphine sulfate** 2-5 mg IV q1h or 0.03-0.05 mg/kg/h IV infusion (100 mg in 250 mL D5W) titrated.

   4. **Propofol (Diprivan):** 50 mcg/kg bolus over 5 min, then 5-50 mcg/kg/min. Titrate in increments of 5 mcg/kg/min.

H. **Paralysis** (with simultaneous amnesia)

   1. **Vecuronium (Norcuron)** 0.1 mg/kg IV, then 0.06 mg/kg/h IV infusion; intermediate acting, maximum neuromuscular blockade within 3-5 min. Half-life 60 min, **OR**

   2. **Cisatracurium (Nimbex)** 0.15 mg/kg IV, then 0.3 mcg/kg/min IV infusion, titrate between 0.5-10 mcg/kg/min. Intermediate acting with

half-life of 25 minutes. Drug of choice for patients with renal or liver impairment, **OR**

3. **Pancuronium (Pavulon)** 0.08 mg/kg IV, then 0.03 mg/kg/h infusion. Long acting, half-life 110 minutes; may cause tachycardia and/or hypertension, **OR**

4. **Atracurium (Tracrium)** 0.5 mg/kg IV, then 0.3-0.6 mg/kg/h infusion, short acting; half-life 20 minutes. Histamine releasing properties may cause bronchospasm and/or hypotension.

5. Monitor level of paralysis with a peripheral nerve stimulator. Adjust neuromuscular blocker dosage to achieve a "train-of-four" (TOF) of 90-95%; if inverse ratio ventilation is being used, maintain TOF at 100%.

I. **Loss at tidal volume:** If a difference between the tidal volume setting and the delivered volume occurs, check for a leak in the ventilator or inspiratory line. Check for a poor seal between the endotracheal tube cuff or malposition of the cuff in the subglottic area. If a chest tube is present, check for air leak.

J. **High peak pressure:** If peak pressure is >40-50, consider bronchospasm, secretion, pneumothorax, ARDS, agitation. Suction the patient and auscultate lungs. Obtain chest radiograph if pneumothorax, pneumonia or ARDS is suspected. Check "plateau pressure" to differentiate airway resistance from compliance causes.

Inverse Ratio Ventilation

1. Indications: ARDS physiology, pAO_2 <60 mm Hg, FIO_2 >0.6, peak airway pressure >45 cm H_2O, or PEEP > 15 cm H_2O. This type of ventilatory support requires heavy sedation and respiratory muscle relaxation.

2. Set oxygen concentration (FIO_2) at 1.0; inspiratory pressure at 1/2 to 1/3 of the peak airway pressure on standard ventilation. Set the inspiration: expiration ratio at 1: 1; set rate at <15 breaths/min. Maintain tidal volume by adjusting inspiratory pressures.

3. Monitor PaO_2, oxygen saturation (by pulse oximetry), $PaCO_2$, end tidal PCO_2, PEEP, mean airway pressure, heart rate, blood pressure, SVO_2, and cardiac output.

4. It SaO_2 remains <0.9, consider increasing I:E ratio (2:1, 3:1), but attempt to keep I:E ratio <2:1. If SaO_2 remains <0.9, increase PEEP or return to conventional mode. If hypotension develops, rule out tension pneumothorax, administer intravascular volume or pressor agents, decrease I:E ratio, or return to conventional ventilation mode.

Ventilator Weaning

I. **Ventilator weaning parameters**
   A. Patient alert and rested
   B. PaO_2 >70 mm Hg on FIO_2 <50%
   C. $PaCO_2$ <50 mm Hg; pH >7.25
   D. Negative Inspiratory Force (NIF) less than -40 cm H_2O
   E. Vital Capacity >10-15 mL/kg (800-1000 mL)
   F. Minute Ventilation (VE) <10 L/min; respirations <24 breaths per min

G. Maximal voluntary minute (MVV) ventilation doubles that of resting minute ventilation (VE).

H. PEEP <5 cm H_2O

I. Tidal volume 5-8 mL/kg

J. Respiratory rate to tidal volume ratio <105

K. No chest wall or cardiovascular instability or excessive secretions

II. Weaning protocols

A. Weaning is considered when patient medical condition (ie, cardiac, pulmonary) status has stabilized.

B. **Indications for termination of weaning trial**
1. PaO_2 falls below 55 mm Hg
2. Acute hypercapnia
3. Deterioration of vital signs or clinical status (arrhythmia)

C. **Rapid T-tube weaning method for short-term (<7 days) ventilator patients without COPD**
1. **Obtain baseline respiratory rate, pulse, blood pressure** and arterial blood gases or oximetry. Discontinue sedation, have the well-rested patient sit in bed or chair. Provide bronchodilators and suctioning if needed.
2. **Attach endotracheal tube** to a T-tube with FiO_2 >10% greater than previous level. Set T-tube flow-by rate to exceed peak inspiratory flow.
3. **Patients who are tried on T-tube trial** should be observed closely for signs of deterioration. After initial 15-minute interval of spontaneous ventilation, resume mechanical ventilation and check oxygen saturation or draw an arterial blood gas sample.
4. **If the 30-minute blood gas is acceptable,** a 60-minute interval may be attempted. After each interval, the patient is placed back on the ventilator for an equal amount of time.
5. **If the 60-minute interval blood gas is acceptable** and the patient is without dyspnea, and if blood gases are acceptable, extubation may be considered.

D. **Pressure support ventilation weaning method**
1. **Pressure support ventilation is initiated at 5-25 cm H_2O.** Set level to maintain the spontaneous tidal volume at 7-15 mL/kg.
2. **Gradually decrease the level of pressure support ventilation** in increments of 3-5 cm H_2O according to the ability of the patient to maintain satisfactory minute ventilation.
3. **Extubation** can be considered at a pressure support ventilation level of 5 cm H_2O provided that the patient can maintain stable respiratory status and blood gasses.

E. **Intermittent mandatory ventilation (IMV) weaning method**
1. **Obtain baseline vital signs and draw baseline arterial blood gases** or pulse oximetry. Discontinue sedation; consider adding pressure support of 10-15 cm H_2O.
2. **Change the ventilator from assist control to IMV mode**; or if already on IMV mode, decrease the rate as follows:
   a. **Patients with no underlying lung disease** and on ventilator for a brief period (<1 week)
      (1) Decrease IMV rate at 30 min intervals by 1-3 breath per min at each step, starting at rate of 8-10 until a rate for zero is reached.
      (2) If each step is tolerated and ABG is adequate (pH >7.3-7.35), extubation may be considered.

        (3) Alternatively: The patient may be watched on minimal support (ie, pressure support with CPAP) after IMV rate of zero is reached. If no deterioration is noted, extubation may be accomplished.

    b. Patients with COPD or prolonged ventilator support (>1 week)

        (1) Begin with IMV at frequency of 8 breath/minute, with tidal volume of 10 mL/kg, with an FiO_2 10% greater than previous setting. Check end-tidal CO_2.

        (2) ABG should be drawn at 30- and 60-minute intervals to check for adequate ventilation and oxygenation. If the patient and/or blood gas deteriorate during weaning trial, then return to previous stable setting.

        (3) Decrease IMV rate in increments of 1-2 breath per hour if the patient is clinical status and blood gases remain stable. Check ABG and saturation one-half hour after a new rate is set.

        (4) If the patient tolerates an IMV rate of zero, decrease the pressure to support in increments of 2-5 cm H_2O per hour until a pressure support of 5 cm H_2O is reached.

        (5) Observe the patient for an additional 24 hours on minimal support before extubation.

  3. Causes of inability to wean patients from ventilators: Bronchospasm, active pulmonary infection, secretions, small endotracheal tube, weakness of respiratory muscle, low cardiac output.

Pulmonary Embolism

More than 500,000 patients are diagnosed with pulmonary emboli annually, resulting in 200,000 deaths. Pulmonary embolism is associated with a mortality rate of 30 percent if untreated. Accurate diagnosis with ventilation/perfusion lung scanning or pulmonary angiography followed by therapy with anticoagulants significantly decreases the mortality rate to 2 to 8 percent.

I. Pathophysiology

  A. Pulmonary emboli usually arise from thrombi in the deep venous system of the lower extremities; however, they may also originate in the pelvic, renal, or upper extremity veins and in the right heart

  B. Risk factors. Patients with pulmonary emboli usually have risk factors for the development of venous thrombosis.

    1. Immobilization.

    2. Surgery within the last three months.

    3. History of venous thromboembolism.

    4. Malignancy is an increased risk associated with obesity (relative risk 2.9), heavy cigarette smoking 25 to 34 cigarettes per day, and hypertension.

  C. Patients with pulmonary emboli without identifiable risk factors (idiopathic or primary venous thromboembolism) may have unsuspected underlying abnormalities that favor the development of thromboembolic disease. Factor V Leiden mutation should be particularly suspected in this setting, being seen in up to 40 percent of cases. High concentrations of factor VIII are present in 11 percent and confer a sixfold risk for venous thromboembolism.

D. When idiopathic venous thromboembolism recurs, occult malignancy should also be suspected, being present in 17 percent of such patients. Venous thromboembolism may be the presenting sign of pancreatic or prostate cancers, breast, lung, uterine, or brain malignancies.

II. **Clinical manifestations.** Sixty-five to 90 percent of pulmonary emboli arise from the lower extremities. However, the majority of patients with pulmonary embolism have no leg symptoms.

A. The most common symptoms are dyspnea (73 percent), pleuritic pain (66 percent), cough (37 percent) and hemoptysis (13 percent).

B. The most common signs are tachypnea (70 percent), rales (51 percent), tachycardia (30 percent), a fourth heart sound (24 percent), and an accentuated pulmonic component of the second heart sound (23 percent).

C. The syndrome of pleuritic pain or hemoptysis without cardiovascular collapse is the most commonly recognized syndrome (65 percent); isolated dyspnea is observed in 22 percent. Circulatory collapse is uncommon (8 percent).

D. Fever, usually with a temperature <102.0°F, occurs in 14 percent of patients with pulmonary embolism.

Frequency of Symptoms and Signs in Pulmonary Embolism			
Symptoms	**Frequency (%)**	**Signs**	**Frequency (%)**
Dyspnea	84	Tachypnea (>16/min)	92
Pleuritic chest pain	74	Rales	58
Apprehension	59	Accentuated S2	53
Cough	53	Tachycardia	44
Hemoptysis	30	Fever (>37.8°C)	43
Sweating	27	Diaphoresis	36
Non-pleuritic chest pain	14	S3 or S4 gallop	34
		Thrombophlebitis	32

III. **Laboratory abnormalities** are nonspecific and include leukocytosis, an increase in the erythrocyte sedimentation rate (ESR), and an elevated serum LDH or AST (SGOT) with a normal serum bilirubin. Arterial blood gases usually reveal hypoxemia, hypocapnia, and respiratory alkalosis.

A. Massive pulmonary embolus with hypotension and respiratory collapse can lead to hypercapnia and a combined respiratory and metabolic acidosis. Additionally, the PaO_2 is between 85 and 105 mm Hg in 18 percent of patients with pulmonary embolism, and up to 6 percent may have a normal alveolar-arterial gradient for oxygen. Arterial blood gas measurements do not play a major role in excluding or establishing the diagnosis of pulmonary embolism.

B. **Serum troponin I and troponin T** are elevated in 30 to 50 percent of patients with a moderate to large pulmonary embolism because of acute right heart overload. Although not useful for diagnosis, elevated troponins are predictive of an adverse prognosis, being associated with marked increases in the incidence of prolonged hypotension and in-hospital mortality.

C. **Electrocardiography** is often abnormal (70 percent); however, the findings are insensitive and nonspecific. The most common abnormalities are nonspecific ST segment and T wave changes (49 percent). The presence of T-wave inversion in the precordial leads may correlate with more severe right ventricular dysfunction.

D. Chest radiography. The most frequent radiographic abnormalities are atelectasis, observed in 69 percent of pulmonary emboli. Pleural effusion is noted in 47 percent.

IV. Diagnostic evaluation

A. Ventilation/perfusion lung scanning is the most frequently used test to aid in the diagnosis of PE in patients in whom a careful physical examination and routine diagnostic tests have failed to reveal a specific diagnosis to explain the pulmonary symptoms.

B. A high probability lung scan indicates a high likelihood of emboli, particularly in patients with a high pretest probability of pulmonary emboli (95 percent). High probability lung scans, however, are not very sensitive for PE (42 percent sensitivity). The majority of pulmonary emboli produce lung scan defects that are intermediate (41 percent of emboli) or low probability (16 percent).

C. Noninvasive lower extremity tests. Noninvasive assessment for deep venous thrombosis may be helpful in the evaluation of patients with intermediate clinical and scan probabilities for pulmonary emboli. Color-flow Doppler with compression ultrasound has high sensitivity (89 to 100 percent) and specificity (89 to 100 percent) for the detection of a first episode of proximal venous thrombosis.

D. D-dimers are detectable at levels greater than 500 ng/mL in nearly all patients with PE. However, an elevated D-dimer concentration is insufficient to establish the diagnosis of PE because such values are nonspecific and are commonly present in hospitalized patients, particularly those with malignancy or recent surgery.

E. Pulmonary angiography. Many patients require angiography to confirm or exclude PE with certainty. Angiography is the definitive diagnostic technique. A negative pulmonary angiogram with magnification excludes clinically relevant pulmonary embolism.

F. Helical CT scanning. Initial reports suggested that the technique had a very high sensitivity, but subsequent studies found sensitivities ranging from 53 to 87 percent.

Pretest Probability of Pulmonary Embolism

High probability - 90 percent
Presence of at least one of three symptoms (sudden onset dyspnea, chest pain, fainting) not otherwise explained and associated with: (1) any two of the following abnormalities: electrocardiographic signs of right ventricular overload, radiographic signs of oligemia, amputation of a hilar artery, or pulmonary consolidation compatible with infarction; (2) any one of the above three radiographic abnormalities.

Intermediate probability - 50 percent
Presence of at least one of the above symptoms, not explained otherwise, but not associated with the above electrocardiographic and radiographic abnormalities, or associated with electrocardiographic signs of right ventricular overload only.

Low probability - 10 percent

Absence of the above three symptoms, or identification of an alternative diagnosis that may account for their presence (eg, exacerbation of COPD, pneumonia, lung edema, myocardial infarction, pneumothorax, and others)

V. **Recommendations.** The combination of clinical assessment, lung scanning, D-dimer testing, and venous ultrasound will confirm or exclude acute pulmonary emboli in many patients.

 A. In patients with suspected pulmonary embolism and leg symptoms, initial testing with venous ultrasonography should be considered.

 B. Anticoagulation can be safely withheld from patients with a low pretest clinical probability and a negative D-dimer.

 C. Anticoagulation also can be safely withheld from patients with low or moderate pretest clinical probability, a non-high probability lung scan, and either negative serial venous ultrasounds or a negative D-dimer.

Weight-based nomogram for intravenous heparin infusion	
Initial dose	80 U/kg bolus, then 18 U/kg per hour
aPTT* <35 sec (<1.2 x control)	80 U/kg bolus, then increase infusion rate by 4 U/kg per hour
aPTT	40 U/kg per hour, then increase infusion by 2 U/kg per hour
aPTT	No change
aPTT	Decrease infusion rate by 2q U/kg per hour
aPTT	Hold infusion 1 hour, then decrease infusion rate by 3 U/kg per hour
*aPTT = activated partial thromboplastin time	

Asthma

Asthma is the most common chronic disease among children. Asthma triggers include viral infections; environmental pollutants, such as tobacco smoke; aspirin, nonsteroidal anti-inflammatory drugs, and sustained exercise, particularly in cold environments.

I. **Diagnosis**

 A. Symptoms of asthma may include episodic complaints of breathing difficulties, seasonal or nighttime cough, prolonged shortness of breath after a respiratory infection, or difficulty sustaining exercise.

 B. Wheezing does not always represent asthma. Wheezing may persist for weeks after an acute bronchitis episode. Patients with chronic obstructive pulmonary disease may have a reversible component superimposed on their fixed obstruction. Etiologic clues include a personal history of allergic disease, such as rhinitis or atopic dermatitis, and a family history of allergic disease.

C. The frequency of daytime and nighttime symptoms, duration of exacerbations and asthma triggers should be assessed.

D. **Physical examination.** Hyperventilation, use of accessory muscles of respiration, audible wheezing, and a prolonged expiratory phase are common. Increased nasal secretions or congestion, polyps, and eczema may be present.

E. **Measurement of lung function.** An increase in the forced expiratory volume in one second (FEV_1) of 12% after treatment with an inhaled beta$_2$ agonist is sufficient to make the diagnosis of asthma. A 12% change in peak expiratory flow rate (PEFR) measured on a peak-flow meter is also diagnostic.

II. Treatment of asthma

A. **Beta$_2$ agonists**

1. Inhaled short-acting beta$_2$-adrenergic agonists are the most effective drugs available for treatment of acute bronchospasm and for prevention of exercise-induced asthma. Levalbuterol (Xopenex), the R-isomer of racemic albuterol, offers no significant advantage over racemic albuterol.

2. **Salmeterol (Serevent)**, a long-acting beta$_2$ agonist, has a relatively slow onset of action and a prolonged effect.

a. Salmeterol should not be used in the treatment of acute bronchospasm. Patients taking salmeterol should use a short-acting beta$_2$ agonist as needed to control acute symptoms. Twice-daily inhalation of salmeterol has been effective for maintenance treatment in combination with inhaled corticosteroids.

b. Fluticasone/Salmeterol (Advair Diskus) is a long-acting beta agonist and corticosteroid combination; dry-powder inhaler [100, 250 or 500 g/puff],1 puff q12h.

3. **Formoterol (Foradil)** is a long-acting beta2 agonist like salmeterol. It should only be used in patients who already take an inhaled corticosteroid. Patients taking formoterol should use a short-acting beta$_2$ agonist as needed to control acute symptoms. For maintenance treatment of asthma in adults and children at least 5 years old, the recommended dosage is 1 puff bid.

4. **Adverse effects of beta$_2$ agonists.** Tachycardia, palpitations, tremor and paradoxical bronchospasm can occur. High doses can cause hypokalemia.

Drugs for Asthma		
Drug	Formulation	Dosage
Inhaled beta$_2$-adrenergic agonists, short-acting		
Albuterol *Proventil* *Proventil-HFA* *Ventolin* *Ventolin Rotacaps*	metered-dose inhaler (90 µg/puff) dry-powder inhaler (200 µg/inhalation)	2 puffs q4-6h PRN 1-2 capsules q4-6h PRN

Drug	Formulation	Dosage
Albuterol *Proventil* multi-dose vials *Ventolin Nebules* *Ventolin*	nebulized	2.5 mg q4-6h PRN
Levalbuterol - *Xopenex*	nebulized	0.63-1.25 mg q6-8h PRN
Inhaled beta2-adrenergic agonist, long-acting		
Formoterol - *Foradil*	oral inhaler (12 µg/capsule)	1 cap q12h via inhaler
Salmeterol *Serevent* *Serevent Diskus*	metered-dose inhaler (21 µg/puff) dry-powder inhaler (50 µg/inhalation)	2 puffs q12h 1 inhalation q12h
Fluticasone/Salmeterol *Advair Diskus*	dry-powder inhaler (100, 250 or 500 µg/puff)	1 puff q12h
Inhaled Corticosteroids		
Beclomethasone dipropionate *Beclovent* *Vanceril* Vanceril Double-Strength	metered-dose inhaler (42 µg/puff) (84 µg/puff)	4-8 puffs bid 2-4 puffs bid
Budesonide *Pulmicort Turbuhaler*	dry-powder inhaler (200 µg/inhalation)	1-2 inhalations bid
Flunisolide - *AeroBid*	metered-dose inhaler (250 µg/puff)	2-4 puffs bid
Fluticasone Flovent *Flovent Rotadisk*	metered-dose inhaler (44, 110 or 220 µg/puff) dry-powder inhaler (50, 100 or 250 µg/inhalation)	2-4 puffs bid (44 µg/puff) 1 inhalation bid (100 µg/inhalation)
Triamcinolone acetonide *Azmacort*	metered-dose inhaler (100 µg/puff)	2 puffs tid-qid or 4 puffs bid
Leukotriene Modifiers		
Montelukast - *Singulair*	tablets	10 mg qhs
Zafirlukast - *Accolate*	tablets	20 mg bid
Zileuton - *Zyflo*	tablets	600 mg qid
Mast Cell Stabilizers		
Cromolyn *Intal*	metered-dose inhaler (800 µg/puff)	2-4 puffs tid-qid

Drug	Formulation	Dosage
Nedocromil *Tilade*	metered-dose inhaler (1.75 mg/puff)	2-4 puffs bid-qid
Phosphodiesterase Inhibitor		
Theophylline *Slo-Bid Gyrocaps, Theo-Dur, Unidur*	extended-release capsules or tablets	100-300 mg bid

B. Inhaled corticosteroids
   1. Regular use of an inhaled corticosteroid can suppress inflammation, decrease bronchial hyperresponsiveness and decrease symptoms. Inhaled corticosteroids are recommended for most patients.
   2. **Adverse effects.** Inhaled corticosteroids are usually free of toxicity. Dose-dependent slowing of linear growth may occur within 6-12 weeks in some children. Decreased bone density, glaucoma and cataract formation have been reported. Churg-Strauss vasculitis has been reported rarely. Dysphonia and oral candidiasis can occur. The use of a spacer device and rinsing the mouth after inhalation decreases the incidence of candidiasis.

C. Leukotriene modifiers
   1. Leukotrienes increase production of mucus and edema of the airway wall, and may cause bronchoconstriction. Montelukast and zafirlukast are leukotriene receptor antagonists. Zileuton inhibits synthesis of leukotrienes.
   2. **Montelukast (Singulair)** is modestly effective for maintenance treatment of intermittent or persistent asthma. It is taken once daily in the evening. It is less effective than inhaled corticosteroids, but addition of montelukast may permit a reduction in corticosteroid dosage. Montelukast added to oral or inhaled corticosteroids can improve symptoms.
   3. **Zafirlukast (Accolate)** is modestly effective for maintenance treatment of mild-to-moderate asthma It is less effective than inhaled corticosteroids. Taking zafirlukast with food markedly decreases its bioavailability. Theophylline can decrease its effect. Zafirlukast increases serum concentrations of oral anticoagulants and may cause bleeding. Infrequent adverse effects include mild headache, gastrointestinal disturbances and increased serum aminotransferase activity. Drug-induced lupus and Churg-Strauss vasculitis have been reported.
   4. **Zileuton (Zyflo)** is modestly effective for maintenance treatment, but it is taken four times a day and patients must be monitored for hepatic toxicity.

D. Cromolyn (Intal) and nedocromil (Tilade)
   1. Cromolyn sodium, an inhibitor of mast cell degranulation, can decrease airway hyperresponsiveness in some patients with asthma. The drug has no bronchodilating activity and is useful only for prophylaxis. Cromolyn has virtually no systemic toxicity.
   2. Nedocromil has similar effects as cromolyn. Both cromolyn and nedocromil are much less effective than inhaled corticosteroids.

E. Theophylline

1. Oral theophylline has a slower onset of action than inhaled beta$_2$ agonists and has limited usefulness for treatment of acute symptoms. It can, however, reduce the frequency and severity of symptoms, especially in nocturnal asthma, and can decrease inhaled corticosteroid requirements.

2. When theophylline is used alone, serum concentrations between 8-12 mcg/mL provide a modest improvement is FEV_1. Serum levels of 15-20 mcg/mL are only minimally more effective and are associated with a higher incidence of cardiovascular adverse events.

F. Oral corticosteroids are the most effective drugs available for acute exacerbations of asthma unresponsive to bronchodilators.

1. Oral corticosteroids decrease symptoms and may prevent an early relapse. Chronic use of oral corticosteroids can cause glucose intolerance, weight gain, increased blood pressure, osteoporosis, cataracts, immunosuppression and decreased growth in children. Alternate-day use of corticosteroids can decrease the incidence of adverse effects, but not of osteoporosis.

2. **Prednisone, prednisolone or methylprednisolone** (Solu-Medrol), 40-60 mg qd; for children, 1-2 mg/kg/day to a maximum of 60 mg/day. Therapy is continued for 3-10 days. The oral steroid dosage does not need to be tapered after short-course "burst" therapy if the patient is receiving inhaled steroid therapy.

Pharmacotherapy for Asthma Based on Disease Classification		
Classification	**Long-term control medications**	**Quick-relief medications**
Mild intermittent		Short-acting beta$_2$ agonist as needed
Mild persistent	Low-dose inhaled corticosteroid or cromolyn sodium (Intal) or nedocromil (Tilade)	Short-acting beta$_2$ agonist as needed
Moderate persistent	Medium-dose inhaled corticosteroid plus a long-acting bronchodilator (long-acting beta$_2$ agonist)	Short-acting beta$_2$ agonist as needed
Severe persistent	High-dose inhaled corticosteroid plus a long-acting bronchodilator and systemic corticosteroid	Short-acting beta$_2$ agonist as needed

III. Management of acute exacerbations

A. High-dose, short-acting beta$_2$ agonists delivered by a metered-dose inhaler with a volume spacer or via a nebulizer remains the mainstay of urgent treatment.

B. Most patients require therapy with systemic corticosteroids to resolve symptoms and prevent relapse. Hospitalization should be considered if the PEFR remains less than 70% of predicted. Patients with a PEFR less than 50% of predicted who exhibit an increasing pCO_2 level and declining mental status are candidates for intubation.

C. Non-invasive ventilation with bilevel positive airway pressure (BIPAP) may be used to relieve the work-of-breathing while awaiting the effects of acute treatment, provided that consciousness and the ability to protect the airway have not been compromised.

Chronic Obstructive Pulmonary Disease

Chronic obstructive pulmonary disease (COPD) is the most common cause of death in the United States and currently kills more than 100,000 Americans each year. COPD is characterized by airflow limitation that is not fully reversible. Airflow limitation is usually both progressive and associated with an abnormal inflammatory response of the lungs to noxious particles or gases.

I. **Pathophysiology**
   A. Airflow obstruction is the result of both small airway disease (obstructive bronchiolitis) and parenchymal destruction (emphysema). Airflow obstruction can be accompanied by partially reversible airways hyperreactivity.
   B. **Alpha-1 antitrypsin (AAT) deficiency** is the only genetic abnormality that predisposes to lung disease similar to COPD. Severe AAT deficiency has a frequency of about 1 in 3,000 live births. These individuals may have liver disease in infancy or in old age, or they may develop AAT-COPD in their thirties or forties, especially if they smoke. About 2 percent of patients with COPD or sustained asthma may have severe AAT deficiency. Persons with known COPD, or asthma with non-remittent airflow obstruction should be screened for AAT deficiency.

II. **Clinical features**
   A. Patients with COPD have usually been smoking at least 20 cigarettes per day for 20 or more years before symptoms develop. Chronic productive cough, sometimes with wheezing, often begins when patients are in their forties.
   B. Dyspnea on effort does not usually begin until the mid sixties or early seventies. Sputum production initially occurs only in the morning. Sputum is usually mucoid but becomes purulent with an exacerbation. Acute chest illnesses may occur intermittently, and are characterized by increased cough, purulent sputum, wheezing, dyspnea, and occasionally fever.
   C. Late in the course of the illness, an exacerbation may cause hypoxemia with cyanosis. Associated findings also include:
      1. Weight loss.
      2. Hypercapnia with more severe hypoxemia in the setting of end-stage disease. Morning headache, which suggests hypercapnia.
      3. Cor pulmonale with right heart failure and edema. These abnormalities can develop in patients with hypoxemia and hypercapnia.
   D. **Physical examination** of the chest early in the disease may show only prolonged expiration and wheezes on forced exhalation. As obstruction progresses, hyperinflation becomes evident, and the anteroposterior diameter of the chest increases. The diaphragm is depressed. Breath sounds are decreased and heart sounds become distant. Coarse crackles may be heard at the lung bases. Wheezes are frequently heard.
      1. Patients with end-stage COPD may lean forward with arms outstretched and weight supported on the palms. Other signs in a patient with end-stage disease may include:
         a. The full use of the accessory respiratory muscles of the neck and shoulder girdle.

    b. Expiration through pursed lips.

    c. Paradoxical retraction of the lower interspaces during inspiration (Hoover's sign).

    d. Cyanosis.

    e. An enlarged, tender liver secondary to right heart failure.

    f. Asterixis due to severe hypercapnia.

E. Plain chest radiography. Emphysema is characterized by over distention of the lungs as indicated on frontal chest radiographs by a low, flat diaphragm and a long, narrow heart shadow. Flattening of the diaphragmatic contour and an increased retrosternal airspace are present on the lateral projection. Rapid tapering of the vascular shadows accompanied by hypertransradiancy of the lungs is a sign of emphysema. Bullae, presenting as radiolucent areas larger than one centimeter in diameter and surrounded by arcuate hairline shadows, are proof of emphysema.

F. Pulmonary function tests are necessary for diagnosing and assessing the severity of airflow obstruction, and are helpful in following its progress. The FEV_1 has less variability than other measurements of airways dynamics. In the mildest degree of airflow obstruction, the FEV_1/FVC ratio falls below 0.70 and the FEV_1 percent predicted is normal. Up to 30 percent of patients have an increase of 15 percent or more in their FEV_1 following inhalation of a beta-agonist.

G. Arterial blood gases reveal mild or moderate hypoxemia without hypercapnia in the early stages. As the disease progresses, hypoxemia becomes more severe and hypercapnia supervenes. The frequency of erythrocytosis increases as arterial PO_2 falls below 55 mm Hg.

H. Sputum examination. In stable chronic bronchitis, sputum is mucoid. During an exacerbation, sputum usually becomes purulent with an influx of neutrophils. The Gram stain usually shows a mixture of organisms. The most frequent pathogens cultured from the sputum are Streptococcus pneumoniae and Haemophilus influenzae.

Diagnosis of chronic obstructive pulmonary disease (COPD)

History
  Smoking history
    Age at initiation
    Average amount smoked per day
    Date when stopped smoking or a current smoker
  Environmental history
  Cough
    Chronic productive cough for at least one quarter of the year for two successive years is the defining characteristic of chronic bronchitis. Sputum, blood or blood streaking in the sputum.
  Wheezing
  Acute chest illnesses
    Frequency of episodes of increased cough and sputum with wheezing.
  Dyspnea
    Amount of effort required to induce uncomfortable breathing.

Physical examination
Chest
The presence of severe emphysema is indicated by: overdistention of the lungs in the stable position; decreased intensity of breath and heart sounds and prolonged expiratory phase.
Wheezes during auscultation on slow or forced breathing and prolongation of forced expiratory time.
Severe disease is indicated by pursed-lip breathing, use of accessory respiratory muscles, retraction of lower interspaces.
Other
Unusual positions to relieve dyspnea at rest.
Digital clubbing suggests the possibility of lung cancer or bronchiectasis.
Mild dependent edema may be seen in the absence of right heart failure.

Differential diagnosis of COPD

Diagnosis	Features
COPD	Onset in mid-life Symptoms slowly progressive Long smoking history Dyspnea during exercise Largely irreversible airflow limitation
Asthma	Onset in childhood Symptoms vary from day to day Symptoms at night/early morning Allergy, rhinitis, and/or eczema also present Family history of asthma Largely reversible airflow limitation
Heart failure	Fine basilar crackles Chest X-ray shows dilated heart, pulmonary edema Pulmonary function tests indicate volume restriction, not airflow limitation
Bronchiectasis	Large volumes of purulent sputum Commonly associated with bacterial infection Coarse crackles/clubbing on auscultation Chest X-ray/CT shows bronchial dilation, bronchial wall thickening
Tuberculosis	Onset all ages Chest X-ray shows lung infiltrate Microbiological confirmation High local prevalence of tuberculosis

Diagnosis	Features
Obliterative bronchiolitis	Onset in younger age, nonsmokers May have history of rheumatoid arthritis or fume exposure CT on expiration shows hypodense areas
Diffuse panbronchiolitis	Most patients are male and non-smokers. Almost all have chronic sinusitis Chest X-ray and HRCT show diffuse small centrilobular nodular opacities and hyperinflation

Classification of Severity of Chronic Obstructive Pulmonary Disease	
Stage	**Characteristics**
0: At risk	Normal spirometry Chronic symptoms (cough, sputum production)
I: Mild COPD	FEV_1/FVC <70 percent FEV_1 $\geq$80 percent predicted With or without chronic symptoms (cough, sputum production)
II: Moderate COPD	FEV_1/FVC <70 percent 30 percent $\leq FEV1$ <80 percent predicted IIA: 50 percent $\leq FEV1$ <80 percent predicted IIB: 30 percent $\leq FEV1$ <50 percent predicted
Severe COPD	FEV_1/FVC <70 percent FEV_1 30 percent predicted or FEV_1 <50 percent predicted plus respiratory failure or clinical signs of right heart failure

III. **Management of Acute Exacerbations of Chronic Obstructive Pulmonary Disease**
   A. **Criteria for hospital admission**. Acute respiratory acidemia and/or worsening hypoxemia justify hospitalization. Specific risk factors for relapse after emergency room (ER) discharge include a prior ER visit within one week, a greater number of doses of nebulized bronchodilator required during the ER visit, use of supplemental oxygen at home, prior relapse after an ER visit, use of aminophylline in the ER, and the use of corticosteroids and/or antibiotics.
   B. **Pharmacologic treatment**
      1. **Inhaled beta-adrenergic agonists,** such as albuterol, are the mainstay of therapy for an acute exacerbation of COPD because of their rapid onset of action and efficacy in producing bronchodilation.
      2. Typical doses of albuterol are 180 mcg (two puffs) by metered dose inhaler, or 500 mcg by nebulizer, given every one to two hours.

3. **Anticholinergic bronchodilators,** such as ipratropium bromide, may be used in combination with beta-adrenergic agonists to produce bronchodilation in excess of that achieved by either agent alone.
   a. **Ipratropium** may be administered during acute exacerbations either by nebulizer (500 mcg every two to four hours), or via MDI (two puffs [36 mcg] every two to four hours with a spacer). Glycopyrrolate is available for nebulized use in COPD (1 to 2 mg every two to four hours).
4. **Parenteral corticosteroids** are frequently used for acute exacerbations of COPD. Methylprednisolone (60 to 125 mg intravenously, two to four times daily) commonly is given.
5. **Antibiotics** are recommended for acute exacerbations of COPD characterized by increased volume and purulence of secretions. A 10-day course of amoxicillin, doxycycline, or trimethoprim-sulfamethoxazole should be prescribed.

Choice of empirical antibiotic therapy for COPD exacerbation	
First-line treatment	**Dosage***
Amoxicillin (Amoxil, Trimox, Wymox)	500 mg tid
Trimethoprim-sulfamethoxazole (Bactrim, Cotrim, Septra)	1 tablet (80/400 mg) bid
Doxycycline	100 mg bid
Erythromycin	250-500 mg qid
Second-line treatment**	
Amoxicillin and clavulanate (Augmentin)	500-875 mg bid
Second- or third-generation cephalosporin (eg, cefuroxime [Ceftin])	250-500 mg bid
Macrolides	
Clarithromycin (Biaxin)	250-500 mg bid
Azithromycin (Zithromax)	500 mg on day 1, then 250 mg qd X 4 days
Quinolones	
Ciprofloxacin (Cipro)	500-750 mg bid
Levofloxacin (Levaquin)***	500 mg qd

*May need adjustment in patients with renal or hepatic insufficiency.
**For patients in whom first-line therapy has failed and those with moderate to severe disease or resistant or gram-negative pathogens.
***Although the newer quinolones have better activity against Streptococcus pneumoniae, ciprofloxacin may be preferable in patients with gram-negative organisms.

6. **Methylxanthines.** Aminophylline and theophylline are not recommended for the management of acute exacerbations of COPD.

C. **Oxygen therapy**
   1. **Supplemental oxygen** should achieve a target PaO_2 of 60 to 65 mm Hg, with a hemoglobin saturation exceeding 90 percent.
   2. **Venturi masks** are the preferred means of oxygen delivery because they permit a precise delivered fraction of inspired oxygen (FiO_2).
   3. **Nasal cannulae** can provide flow rates up to 6 L/min with an associated FiO_2 of approximately 44 percent. Nasal cannulae are also more comfortable for the patient and permit oral feedings.
   4. **Facemasks** can be used when higher inspired concentrations of oxygen are needed. Simple facemasks using flow rates of 6 to 10 L/min provide an FiO_2 up to 55 percent.
   5. **Non-rebreather masks** with a reservoir, one-way valves, and a tight face seal can deliver an inspired oxygen concentration up to 90 percent.

D. **Mechanical ventilation.** Patients with life-threatening respiratory failure require ventilatory assistance.
   1. Noninvasive positive pressure ventilation (NIPPV) is effective and less morbid than intubation for selected patients with acute exacerbations of COPD. Early use of NIPPV is recommended when each of the following is present:
      a. Respiratory distress with moderate-to-severe dyspnea.
      b. pH less than 7.35 or $PaCO_2$ above 45 mm Hg.
      c. Respiratory rate of 25/minute or greater.
   2. NIPPV is contraindicated in the presence of cardiovascular instability (eg, hypotension, serious dysrhythmias, myocardial ischemia), craniofacial trauma or burns, inability to protect the airway, or when indications for emergent intubation are present. Approximately 26 to 31 percent of patients initially treated with NIPPV ultimately require intubation and mechanical ventilation.

IV. **Management of Stable Chronic Obstructive Pulmonary Disease (COPD).**
   A. Determination of FEV_1 and FVC by spirometry is the only reliable method of detecting mild airflow limitation and is therefore mandatory for all adults with a history of cigarette smoking. Spirometry is useful to monitor the course of the disease. A plain chest radiograph is indicated to exclude the presence of other disorders associated with airflow limitation.
   B. **Bronchodilators.** Bronchodilators can improve symptoms and reduce airflow limitation in patients with COPD. Use of a metered dose inhaler (MDI) results in a bronchodilator response equivalent to that of a nebulizer. Nebulizer therapy may still be necessary if dyspnea and severe bronchospasm during impair proper MDI technique.
      1. **Selective beta-2 agonists** are the sympathomimetic agents of choice. Beta-2 agonists can cause tremor and a reflex tachycardia. Hypokalemia can also occur and should be monitored in patients at risk.

Scheduled use of short-acting beta-2 agonists, such as albuterol, does not offer advantages over as-needed use.

C. **Anticholinergic bronchodilators,** such as inhaled ipratropium, are first-line treatments for COPD. The long-acting inhaled anticholinergic agent, tiotropium, confers longer bronchodilation than ipratropium and lessens the frequency of acute exacerbations in patients with moderate COPD. The effects of anticholinergics and beta-2 agonists are additive. Combination therapy may be simplified with a metered dose inhaler that delivers a combination of ipratropium and albuterol.

1. The recommended dose of ipratropium (2 puffs qid) is suboptimal; higher doses (3 to 6 puffs) provide additional benefit without significant side effects.

Therapy at each stage of COPD			
Stage	**Characteristics**	**Recommended treatments**	
ALL		Avoidance of risk factor(s) Influenza vaccination	
0: At risk	Chronic symptoms (cough, sputum) Exposure to risk factor(s)		
I: Mild COPD	FEV_1/FVC <70 percent $FEV_1 \geq 80$ percent predicted with or without symptoms	Short-acting bronchodilator when needed	
II: Moderate COPD	IIA		
	FEV_1/FVC <70 percent 50 percent $\leq FEV_1$ <80 percent With or without symptoms	Regular treatment with one or more broncho-dialtors Rehabilitation	Inhaled glucorticosteroids if significant symptoms and lung function response

	IIB		
	FEV$_1$/FVC <70 percent 50 percent $\leq$FEV$_1$ <50 percent With our without symptoms	Regular treatment with one or more bronchodilators Rehabilitation	Inhaled glucorticosteroids if significant symptoms and lung function response or if repeated exacerbations
III: Severe COPD	FEV$_1$/FVC <70 percent FEV$_1$ <30 percent predicted or presence of respiratory or right heart failure	Regular treatment with one or more bronchodilators Inhaled glucorticosteroids if significant symptoms and lung function response or if repeated exacerbations Treatment of complications Rehabilitation Long-term oxygen therapy if respiratory failure Surgical treatments	

D. **Theophylline** provides clear benefits to some patients with COPD. Theophylline decreases dyspnea and improves arterial blood gases, FEV$_1$, FVC, and respiratory muscle function. Theophylline also has pulmonary vasodilator and cardiac inotropic effects. Patients with COPD can be adequately treated with serum levels in the 8 to 12 mcg/mL range. A long-acting preparation at night may reduce the nocturnal dyspnea.

E. **Supplemental oxygen**
   1. Arterial blood gases or pulse oximetry is useful for detecting hypoxemia and hypercapnia. Oxygen therapy in ambulatory outpatients has physiologic and symptomatic benefits and prolongs life.
   2. Noninvasive ventilatory support may be utilized in the treatment of acute and chronic respiratory insufficiency.

F. **Corticosteroids.** Twenty percent of stable patients with COPD demonstrate objective improvement in airflow with oral corticosteroids. Chronic steroid therapy should be considered only in patients who have continued symptoms despite maximal therapy with other agents. Only patients with documented improvement in airflow during a trial should be considered for long-term therapy. Alternate day or inhaled steroids should be considered in steroid-responding patients.

G. **Prevention and treatment of infection.** Pneumococcal vaccination is recommended for all patients with COPD, with revaccination after more than five years for those at risk for significant declines in immune function.
   1. Annual influenza vaccine is recommended in patients with COPD.
   2. Antiviral agents should be considered in nonimmunized patients at high risk for contracting influenza.

3. Antibiotics have been shown to be beneficial in the treatment of acute infectious exacerbations of COPD. Examination of the sputum gram stain for purulence may be of help in determining the need for antibiotics.

H. **Surgical management**
   1. **Lung volume reduction surgery (LVRS)** is recommended in patients with upper lobe predominant disease and low exercise capacity.
   2. **Indications for lung transplantation**
      a. FEV_1 is <25 percent of predicted, **OR**
      b. $PaCO_2$ is >55 mm Hg (7.3 kPa), **OR**
      c. Cor pulmonale is present.
      d. Candidates must be under 65 years of age, not have dysfunction of major organs other than the lung, and not have active or recent malignancy or infection with HIV, hepatitis B, or hepatitis C viruses.

Pleural Effusion

I. **Indications.** The indication for diagnostic thoracentesis is the new finding of a pleural effusion.
   A. **Pre-thoracentesis chest x-ray:** A bilateral decubitus x-ray should be obtained before the thoracentesis. Thoracentesis is safe when fluid freely layers out and is greater than 10 mm in depth on the decubitus film.
   B. **Labs:** CBC, ABG, SMA 12, protein, albumin, amylase, rheumatoid factor, ANA, ESR. INR/PTT, UA. Chest x-ray PA & LAT repeat after thoracentesis, bilateral decubitus, ECG.
   C. **Pleural fluid analysis:**
      1. **Tube 1.** LDH, protein, amylase, triglyceride, glucose (10 mL).
      2. **Tube 2.** Gram stain, C&S, AFB, fungal C&S, (20-60 mL, heparinized).
      3. **Tube 3.** Cell count and differential (5-10 mL, EDTA).
      4. **Tube 4.** Antigen tests for S. pneumoniae, H. influenza (25-50 mL, heparinized).
      5. **Syringe.** pH (2 mL collected anaerobically, heparinized on ice).
      6. **Bottle.** Cytology.

Differential Diagnosis		
Pleural Fluid Parameters	**Transudate**	**Exudate**
LDH (IU)	<200	>200
Pleural LDH/serum LDH	<0.6	>0.6
Total protein (g/dL)	<3.0	>3.0
Pleural Protein/serum Protein	<0.5	>0.5

II. Separation of transudates and exudates

A. Transudates. Transudates are largely caused by imbalances in hydrostatic and oncotic pressures in the chest. However, they can also result from movement of fluid from the peritoneal or retroperitoneal spaces, or from iatrogenic causes, such as crystalloid infusion into a central venous catheter that has migrated.

B. Exudates. Exudative pleural effusions are caused by infection, malignancy, immunologic responses, lymphatic abnormalities, noninfectious inflammation, iatrogenic causes, and movement of fluid from below the diaphragm. Exudates result from pleural and lung inflammation or from impaired lymphatic drainage of the pleural space. Exudates can also result from movement of fluid from the peritoneal space, as seen with pancreatitis, chylous ascites, and peritoneal carcinomatosis.

Diagnoses that can be established definitively by pleural fluid analysis	
Disease	**Diagnostic pleural fluid test**
Empyema	Observation (pus, putrid odor); culture
Malignancy	Positive cytology
Lupus pleuritis	LE cells present; pleural fluid serum ANA >1.0
Tuberculous pleurisy	Positive AFB stain, culture
Esophageal rupture	High salivary amylase, pleural fluid acidosis (often as low as 6.00)
fungal pleurisy	Positive KOH stain, culture
Chylothorax	Triglycerides (>110 mg/dL); lipoprotein electrophoresis (chylomicrons)
Hemothorax	Hematocrit (pleural fluid/blood >0.5)
Urinothorax	Creatinine (pleural fluid/serum >1.0)
Peritoneal dialysis	Protein (<1g/dL); glucose (300 to 400 mg/dL)
Extravascular migration of central venous catheter	Observation (milky if lipids are infused); pleural fluid/serum glucose >1.0
Rheumatoid pleurisy	Characteristic cytology

C. Diagnostic criteria. The most practical method of separating transudates and exudates is measurement of serum and pleural fluid protein and LDH. If at least one of the following three criteria is present, the fluid is virtually always an exudate; if none is present, the fluid is virtually always a transudate:

1. Pleural fluid protein/serum protein ratio greater than 0.5.
2. Pleural fluid LDH/serum LDH ratio greater than 0.6.
3. Pleural fluid LDH greater than two thirds the upper limits of normal of the serum LDH.

Causes of Transudative Pleural Effusions	
Effusion always transudative	
Congestive heart failure	Urinothorax
Hepatic hydrothorax	Atelectasis
Nephrotic syndrome	Constrictive pericarditis
Peritoneal dialysis	Trapped lung
Hypoalbuminemia	Superior vena caval obstruction
Classic exudates that can be transudates	
Malignancy	Sarcoidosis
Pulmonary embolism	Hypothyroid pleural effusion

D. An exudate is best determined by any one of the following:
1. Pleural fluid protein >2.9 g/dL
2. Pleural fluid cholesterol >45 mg/dL
3. Pleural fluid LDH >60 percent of upper limits of normal serum value

Causes of exudative pleural effusions	
Infectious	**Increased negative intrapleural pressure**
Bacterial pneumonia	
Tuberculous pleurisy	Atelectasis
Parasites	Trapped lung
Fungal disease	Cholesterol effusion
Atypical pneumonia (viral, mycoplasma)	
Nocardia, Actinomyces	
Subphrenic abscess	
Hepatic abscess	
Splenic abscess	
Hepatitis	
Spontaneous esophageal rupture	
Iatrogenic	**Endocrine dysfunction**
Drug-induced	Hypothyroidism
Esophageal perforation	Ovarian hyperstimulation syndrome
Esophageal sclerotherapy	
Central venous catheter misplacement/migration	
Enteral feeding tube in pleural space	
Malignancy	**Lymphatic abnormalities**
Carcinoma	Malignancy
Lymphoma	Chylothorax
Mesothelioma	Yellow nail syndrome
Leukemia	Lymphangiomyomatosis
Chylothorax	Lymphangiectasia
Paraproteinemia (multiple myeloma, Waldenstrom's macroglobulinemia)	

Other inflammatory disorders	Movement of fluid from abdomen to pleural space
Pancreatitis (acute, chronic)	Pancreatitis
Benign asbestos pleural effusion	Pancreatic pseudocyst
Pulmonary embolism	Meigs' syndrome
Radiation therapy	Carcinoma
Uremic pleurisy	Chylous ascites
Sarcoidosis	Subphrenic abscess
Postcardiac injury syndrome	Hepatic abscess (bacterial, amebic)
Hemothorax	Splenic abscess, infarction
ARDS	

III. Chemical analysis

A. Pleural fluid protein and LDH

1. Most transudates have absolute total protein concentrations below 3.0 g/dL; however, acute diuresis in congestive heart failure can elevate protein levels into the exudative range.

2. Tuberculous pleural effusions virtually always have total protein concentrations above 4.0 g/dL. When pleural fluid protein concentrations are in the 7.0 to 8.0 g/dL range, Waldenstrom's macroglobulinemia and multiple myeloma should be considered.

3. Pleural fluid LDH levels above 1000 IU/L are found in empyema, rheumatoid pleurisy, and pleural paragonimiasis, and are sometimes observed with malignancy. Pleural fluid secondary to Pneumocystis carinii pneumonia has a pleural fluid/serum LDH ratio greater than 1.0 and a pleural fluid/serum protein ratio of less than 0.5.

B. Pleural fluid glucose.
A low pleural fluid glucose concentration (less than 60 mg/dL), or a pleural fluid/serum glucose ratio less than 0.5) narrows the differential diagnosis of the exudate to the following possibilities:

1. Rheumatoid pleurisy
2. Complicated parapneumonic effusion or empyema
3. Malignant effusion
4. Tuberculous pleurisy
5. Lupus pleuritis
6. Esophageal rupture

C.
All transudates and all other exudates have pleural fluid glucose concentrations similar to that of blood glucose. The lowest glucose concentrations are found in rheumatoid pleurisy and empyema, with glucose being undetectable in some cases. In comparison, when the glucose concentration is low in tuberculous pleurisy, lupus pleuritis, and malignancy, it usually falls into the range of 30 to 50 mg/dL.

D. Pleural fluid pH.
Pleural fluid pH should always be measured in a blood gas machine. A pleural fluid pH below 7.30 with a normal arterial blood pH is found with the same diagnoses associated with low pleural fluid glucose concentrations. The pH of normal pleural fluid is approximately 7.60. Transudates have a pleural fluid pH in the 7.40 to 7.55 range, while the majority of exudates range from 7.30 to 7.45.

E. Pleural fluid amylase.
The finding of an amylase-rich pleural effusion, defined as either a pleural fluid amylase greater than the upper limits of normal for serum amylase or a pleural fluid to serum amylase ratio

greater than 1.0, narrows the differential diagnosis of an exudative effusion to the following major possibilities:

1. Acute pancreatitis
2. Chronic pancreatic pleural effusion
3. Esophageal rupture
4. Malignancy
5. Other rare causes of an amylase-rich pleural effusion include pneumonia, ruptured ectopic pregnancy, hydronephrosis, and cirrhosis. Pancreatic disease is associated with pancreatic isoenzymes, while malignancy and esophageal rupture are characterized by a predominance of salivary isoenzymes.

IV. Pleural fluid nucleated cells
   A. Counts above 50,000/µL are usually found only in complicated parapneumonic effusions, including empyema.
   B. Exudative effusions from bacterial pneumonia, acute pancreatitis, and lupus pleuritis usually have total nucleated cell counts above 10,000/µL.
   C. Chronic exudates, typified by tuberculous pleurisy and malignancy, typically have nucleated cell counts below 5000/µL.
   D. **Pleural fluid lymphocytosis.** Pleural fluid lymphocytosis, particularly with lymphocyte counts representing 85 to 95 percent of the total nucleated cells, suggests tuberculous pleurisy, lymphoma, sarcoidosis, chronic rheumatoid pleurisy, yellow nail syndrome, or chylothorax. Carcinomatous pleural effusions will be lymphocyte predominant in over one-half of cases; however, the percentage of lymphocytes is usually between 50 and 70 percent.
   E. **Pleural fluid eosinophilia.** Pleural fluid eosinophilia (pleural fluid eosinophils representing more than 10 percent of the total nucleated cells) usually suggests a benign, self-limited disease, and is commonly associated with air or blood in the pleural space. The differential diagnosis of pleural fluid eosinophilia includes:
      1. Pneumothorax
      2. Hemothorax
      3. Pulmonary infarction
      4. Benign asbestos pleural effusion
      5. Parasitic disease
      6. Fungal infection (coccidioidomycosis, cryptococcosis, histoplasmosis)
      7. Drugs
      8. Malignancy (carcinoma, lymphoma)
      9. Pleural fluid eosinophilia appears to be rare with tuberculous pleurisy on the initial thoracentesis
   F. **Mesothelial cells** are found in small numbers in normal pleural fluid, are prominent in transudative pleural effusions, and are variable in exudative effusions. Tuberculosis is unlikely if there are more than five percent mesothelial cells.
   G. **Treatment:** Chest tube drainage is indicated for complicated parapneumonic effusions (pH <7.10, glucose <40 mEq/dL, LDH >1000 IU/L) and frank empyema.

References: See page 168.

Trauma

Blanding U. Jones, MD

Pneumothorax

I. Management of pneumothorax

A. Small primary spontaneous pneumothorax (<10-15%): (not associated with underlying pulmonary diseases). If the patient is not dyspneic

1. Observe for 4-8 hours and repeat a chest x-ray.
2. If the pneumothorax does not increase in size and the patient remains asymptomatic, consider discharge home with instructions to rest and curtail all strenuous activities. The patient should return if there is an increase in dyspnea or recurrence of chest pain.

B. Secondary spontaneous pneumothorax (associated with underlying pulmonary pathology, emphysema) or primary spontaneous pneumothorax >15%, or if patient is symptomatic.

1. Give high-flow oxygen by nasal cannula. A needle thoracotomy should be placed at the anterior, second intercostal space in the midclavicular line.
2. Anesthetize and prep the area, then insert a 16-gauge needle with an internal catheter and a 60 mL syringe, attached via a 3-way stopcock. Aspirate until no more air is aspirated. If no additional air can be aspirated, and the volume of aspirated air is <4 liters, occlude the catheter and observe for 4 hours.
3. If symptoms abate and chest-x-ray does not show recurrence of the pneumothorax, the catheter can be removed, and the patient can be discharged home with instructions.
4. If the aspirated air is >4 liters and additional air is aspirated without resistance, this represents an active bronchopleural fistula with continued air leak. Admission is required for insertion of a chest tube.

C. Traumatic pneumothorax associated with a penetrating injury, hemothorax, mechanical ventilation, tension pneumothorax, or if pneumothorax does not resolve after needle aspiration: Give high-flow oxygen and insert a chest tube. Do not delay the management of a tension pneumothorax until radiographic confirmation; insert needle thoracotomy or chest tube immediately.

D. Iatrogenic pneumothorax

1. Iatrogenic pneumothoraces include lung puncture caused by thoracentesis or central line placement.
2. Administer oxygen by nasal cannula.
3. **If the pneumothorax is less than 10% and the patient is asymptomatic,** observe and repeat chest x-ray in 4 hours. If unchanged, manage expectantly with close follow-up, and repeat chest x-ray in 24 hours.
4. **If the pneumothorax is more than 10% and/or the patient is symptomatic,** perform a tube thoracostomy under negative pressure.

II. Technique of chest tube insertion

A. Place patient in supine position, with involved side elevated 20 degrees. Abduct the arm to 90 degrees. The usual site is the fourth or fifth intercostal space, between the mid-axillary and anterior axillary line (drainage of air or free fluid). The point at which the anterior axillary fold meets the chest wall is a useful guide. Alternatively, the second or third intercostal space, in the midclavicular line, may be used for pneumothorax drainage alone (air only).

B. Cleanse the skin with Betadine iodine solution, and drape the field. Determine the intrathoracic tube distance (lateral chest wall to the apices), and mark the length of tube with a clamp.

C. Infiltrate 1% lidocaine into the skin, subcutaneous tissues, intercostal muscles, periosteum, and pleura using a 25-gauge needle. Use a scalpel to make a transverse skin incision, 2 centimeters wide, located over the rib, just inferior to the interspace where the tube will penetrate the chest wall.

D. Use a Kelly clamp to bluntly dissect a subcutaneous tunnel from the skin incision, extending just over the superior margin of the lower rib. Avoid the nerve, artery and vein located at the upper margin of the intercostal space.

E. Penetrate the pleura with the clamp, and open the pleura 1 centimeter. With a gloved finger, explore the subcutaneous tunnel, and palpate the lung medially. Exclude possible abdominal penetration, and ensure correct location within pleural space; use finger to remove any local pleural adhesions.

F. Use the Kelly clamp to grasp the tip of the thoracostomy tube (36 F, internal diameter 12 mm), and direct it into the pleural space in a posterior, superior direction for pneumothorax evacuation. Direct the tube inferiorly for pleural fluid removal. Guide the tube into the pleural space until the last hole is inside the pleural space and not inside the subcutaneous tissue.

G. Attach the tube to a underwater seal apparatus containing sterile normal saline, and adjust to 20 cm H_2O of negative pressure, or attach to suction if leak is severe. Suture the tube to the skin of the chest wall using O silk. Apply Vaseline gauze, 4 x 4 gauze sponges, and elastic tape. Obtain a chest x-ray to verify correct placement and evaluate reexpansion of the lung.

Tension Pneumothorax

I. Clinical evaluation

A. **Clinical signs:** Severe hemodynamic and/or respiratory compromise; contralaterally deviated trachea; decreased or absent breath sounds and hyperresonance to percussion on the affected side; jugular venous distention, asymmetrical chest wall motion with respiration.

B. **Radiologic signs:** Flattening or inversion of the ipsilateral hemidiaphragm; contralateral shifting of the mediastinum; flattening of the cardio-mediastinal contour and spreading of the ribs on the ipsilateral side.

II. Acute management

A. A temporary large-bore IV catheter may be inserted into the ipsilateral pleural space, at the level of the second intercostal space at the midclavicular line until the chest tube is placed.

B. A chest tube should be placed emergently.

C. Draw blood for CBC, INR, PTT, type and cross-matching, chem 7, toxicology screen.

D. Send pleural fluid for hematocrit, amylase and pH (to rule out esophageal rupture).

E. **Indications for cardiothoracic exploration:** Severe or persistent hemodynamic instability despite aggressive fluid resuscitation, persistent active blood loss from chest tube, more than 200 cc/hr for 3 consecutive hours, or ≥ 1 1/2 L of acute blood loss after chest tube placement.

Cardiac Tamponade

I. General considerations
A. Cardiac tamponade occurs most commonly secondary to penetrating injuries.
B. **Beck's Triad:** Venous pressure elevation, drop in the arterial pressure, muffled heart sounds. Other signs include enlarged cardiac silhouette on chest x-ray; signs and symptoms of hypovolemic shock; pulseless electrical activity, decreased voltage on ECG.
C. Kussmaul's sign is characterized by a rise in venous pressure with inspiration. Pulsus paradoxus or elevated venous pressure may be absent when associated with hypovolemia.

II. Management
A. Pericardiocentesis is indicated if the patient is unresponsive to resuscitation measures for hypovolemic shock, or if there is a high likelihood of injury to the myocardium or one of the great vessels.
B. All patients who have a positive pericardiocentesis (recovery of non-clotting blood) because of trauma, require an open thoracotomy with inspection of the myocardium and the great vessels.
C. Rule out other causes of cardiac tamponade such as pericarditis, penetration of central line through the vena cava, atrium, or ventricle, or infection.
D. Consider other causes of hemodynamic instability that may mimic cardiac tamponade (tension pneumothorax, massive pulmonary embolism, shock secondary to massive hemothorax).

Pericardiocentesis

I. General considerations
A. If acute cardiac tamponade with hemodynamic instability is suspected, emergency pericardiocentesis should be performed; infusion of Ringer's lactate, crystalloid, colloid and/or blood may provide temporizing measures.

II. Management
A. Protect airway and administer oxygen. If patient can be stabilized, pericardiocentesis should be performed in the operating room or catheter lab. The para-xiphoid approach is used for pericardiocentesis.
B. **Place patient in supine position** with chest elevated at 30-45 degrees, then cleanse and drape peri-xiphoid area. Infiltrate lidocaine 1% with epinephrine (if time permits) into skin and deep tissues.
C. **Attach a long, large bore (12-18 cm, 16-18 gauge), short bevel cardiac needle** to a 50 cc syringe with a 3-way stop cock. Use an alligator clip to attach a V-lead of the ECG to the metal of the needle.
D. **Advance the needle** just below costal margin, immediately to the left and inferior to the xiphoid process. Apply suction to the syringe while

advancing the needle slowly at a 45 -degree horizontal angle towards the mid point of the left clavicle.

E. **As the needle penetrates** the pericardium, resistance will be felt, and a "popping" sensation will be noted.

F. **Monitor the ECG** for ST segment elevation (indicating ventricular heart muscle contact); or PR segment elevation (indicating atrial epicardial contact). After the needle comes in contact with the epicardium, withdraw the needle slightly. Ectopic ventricular beats are associated with cardiac penetration.

G. Aspirate as much blood as possible. Blood from the pericardial space usually will not clot. Blood, inadvertently, drawn from inside the ventricles or atrium usually will clot. If fluid is not obtained, redirect the needle more towards the head. Stabilize the needle by attaching a hemostat or Kelly clamp.

H. Consider emergency thoracotomy to determine the cause of hemopericardium (especially if active bleeding). If the patient does not improve, consider other problems that may resemble tamponade, such as tension pneumothorax, pulmonary embolism, or shock secondary to massive hemothorax.

References: See page 168.

Hematologic Disorders

Thomas Vovan, MD

Transfusion Reactions

I. **Acute hemolytic transfusion reaction**
   A. Transfusion reactions are rare and most commonly associated with ABO incompatibility, usually related to a clerical error. Early symptoms include sudden onset of anxiety, flushing, tachycardia, and hypotension. Chest and back pain, fever, and dyspnea are common.
   B. Life-threatening manifestations include vascular collapse (shock), renal failure, bronchospasm, and disseminated intravascular coagulation.
   C. Hemoglobinuria, and hemoglobinemia occurs because of intravascular red cell lysis.
   D. The direct antiglobulin test (direct Coombs test) is positive. The severity of reaction is usually related to the volume of RBCs infused.
   E. **Management**
      1. The transfusion should be discontinued immediately, and the unused donor blood and a sample of recipient's venous blood should be sent for retyping and repeat cross match, including a direct and indirect Coombs test.
      2. Urine analysis should be checked for free hemoglobin and centrifuged plasma for pink coloration (indicating free hemoglobin).
      3. Hypotension should be treated with normal saline. Vasopressors may be used if volume replacement alone is inadequate to maintain blood pressure.
      4. Maintain adequate renal perfusion with volume replacement. Furosemide may be used to maintain urine output after adequate volume replacement has been achieved.
      5. Monitor INR/PTT, platelets, fibrinogen, and fibrin degradation products for evidence of disseminated intravascular coagulation. Replace required clotting factors with fresh frozen plasma, platelets, and/or cryoprecipitate.

II. **Febrile transfusion reaction (nonhemolytic)**
   A. Febrile transfusion reactions occur in 0.5-3% of transfusions. It is most commonly seen in patients receiving multiple transfusions. Chills develop, followed by fever, usually during or within a few hours of transfusion. This reaction may be severe but is usually mild and self limited.
   B. **Management**
      1. Symptomatic and supportive care should be provided with acetaminophen and diphenhydramine. Meperidine 50 mg IV is useful in treating chills. A WBC filter should be used for the any subsequent transfusions.
      2. More serious transfusion reactions must be excluded (eg, acute hemolytic reaction or bacterial contamination of donor blood).

III. **Transfusion-related noncardiogenic pulmonary edema**
   A. This reaction is characterized by sudden development of severe respiratory distress, associated with fever, chills, chest pain, and hypotension.
   B. Chest radiograph demonstrates diffuse pulmonary edema. This reaction may be severe and life threatening but generally resolves within 48 hours.

C. Management
1. Treatment of pulmonary edema and hypoxemia may include mechanical ventilatory support and hemodynamic monitoring.
2. Diuretics are useful only if fluid overload is present. Use a WBC filter should be used for any subsequent transfusions.

Disseminated Intravascular Coagulation

I. Clinical manifestations
A. Disseminated intravascular coagulation (DIC) is manifest by generalized ecchymosis and petechiae, bleeding from peripheral IV sites, central catheters, surgical wounds, and oozing from gums.
B. Gastrointestinal and urinary tract bleeding are frequently encountered. Grayish discoloration or cyanosis of the distal fingers, toes, or ears may occur because of intravascular thrombosis. Large, sharply demarcated, ecchymotic areas may be seen as a result of thrombosis.

II. Diagnosis
A. Fibrin degradation products are the most sensitive screening test for DIC; however, no single laboratory parameter is diagnostic of DIC.
B. **Peripheral smear:** Evidence of microangiopathic hemolysis, with schistocytes and thrombocytopenia, is often present. A persistently normal platelet count nearly excludes the diagnosis of acute DIC.
C. **Coagulation studies:** INR, PTT, and thrombin time are generally prolonged. Fibrinogen levels are usually depleted (<150 mg/dL). Fibrin degradation products (>10 mg/dL) and D-dimer is elevated (>0.5 mg/dL).

III. Management of disseminated intravascular coagulation
A. The primary underlying precipitating condition (eg, sepsis) should be treated. Severe DIC with hypocoagulability may be treated with replacement of clotting factors. Hypercoagulability is managed with heparin.
B. Severe hemorrhage and shock is managed with fluids and red blood cell transfusions.
C. **If the patient is at high risk of bleeding or actively bleeding with DIC:** Replace fibrinogen with 10 units of cryoprecipitate. Replace clotting factors with 2-4 units of fresh frozen plasma. Replace platelets with platelet pheresis.
D. **If factor replacement therapy is transfused,** fibrinogen and platelet levels should be obtained 30-60 minutes post-transfusion and every 4-6 hours thereafter to determine the efficacy of therapy. Each unit of platelets should increase the platelet count by 5000-10,000/mcL. Each unit of cryoprecipitate should increase the fibrinogen level by 5-10 mg/dL.
E. **Heparin**
1. Indications for heparin include evidence of fibrin deposition (ie, dermal necrosis, acral ischemia, venous thromboembolism). Heparin is used when the coagulopathy is believed to be secondary to a retained, dead fetus, amniotic fluid embolus, giant hemangioma, aortic aneurysm, solid tumors, or promyelocytic leukemia. Heparin is also used when clotting factors cannot be corrected with replacement therapy alone.
2. Heparin therapy is initiated at a relatively low dose (5-10 U/kg/hr) by continuous IV infusion without a bolus. Coagulation parameters must then be followed to guide therapy. The heparin dose may be increased by 2.5 U/kg/hr until the desired effect is achieved.

Thrombolytic-associated Bleeding

I. **Clinical presentation**: Post-fibrinolysis hemorrhage may present as a sudden neurologic deficit (intracranial bleeding), massive GI bleeding, progressive back pain accompanied by hypotension (retroperitoneal bleeding), or a gradual decline in hemoglobin without overt evidence of bleeding.

II. **Laboratory evaluation**
   A. Low fibrinogen (<100 mg/dL) and elevated fibrin degradation products confirm the presence of a lytic state. Elevated thrombin time and PTT may suggest a persistent lytic state; however, both are prolonged in the presence of heparin. Prolonged reptilase time identifies the persistent lytic state in the presence of heparin.
   B. Depleted fibrinogen in the fibrinolytic state will be reflected by an elevated PTT, thrombin time, or reptilase time. The post-transfusion fibrinogen level is a useful indicator of response to replacement therapy.
   C. The bleeding time may be a helpful guide to platelet replacement therapy if the patient has persistent bleeding despite factor replacement with cryoprecipitate and fresh frozen plasma.

III. **Management**
   A. Discontinue thrombolytics, aspirin, and heparin immediately, and consider protamine reversal of heparin and cryoprecipitate to replenish fibrinogen.
   B. Place two large-bore IV catheters for volume replacement. If possible, apply local pressure to bleeding sites. Blood specimens should be sent for INR/PTT, fibrinogen, and thrombin time. Reptilase time should be checked if the patient is also receiving heparin. Patient's blood should be typed and crossed because urgent transfusion may be needed.
   C. **Transfusion**
      1. Cryoprecipitate (10 units over 10 minutes) should be transfused to correct the lytic state. Transfusions may be repeated until the fibrinogen level is above 100 mg/dL or hemostasis is achieved. Cryoprecipitate is rich in fibrinogen and factor VIII.
      2. Fresh frozen plasma transfusion is also important for replacement of factor VIII and V. If bleeding persists after cryoprecipitate and FFP replacement, check a bleeding time and consider platelet transfusion if bleeding time is greater than 9 minutes. If bleeding time is less than 9 minutes, then antifibrinolytic drugs may be warranted.
   D. **Antifibrinolytic agents**
      1. Aminocaproic acid (EACA) inhibits the conversion of plasminogen to plasmin. It is used when replacement of blood products are not sufficient to attain hemostasis.
      2. Loading dose: 5 g or 0.1 g/kg IV infused in 250 cc NS over 30-60 min, followed by continuous infusion at 0.5-2.0 g/h until bleeding is controlled. Use with caution in upper urinary tract bleeding because of the potential for obstruction.

References: See page 168.

Infectious Diseases

Guy Foster, MD
Farhad Mazdisnian, MD
Michael Krutzik, MD
Georgina Heal, MD

Bacterial Meningitis

Meningitis is an infection of the meninges and the cerebrospinal fluid (CSF) of the subarachnoid space and the cerebral ventricles. Meningitis is one of the ten most common infectious causes of death. Neurologic sequelae are common among survivors.

I. **Epidemiology**
   A. **Causative organisms in adults**
      1. Up to age 60, S. pneumoniae is responsible for 60 percent of cases, followed by N. meningitidis (20 percent), H. influenzae (10 percent), L. monocytogenes (6 percent), and group B streptococcus (4 percent).
      2. Age 60 and above, almost 70 percent of cases are caused by S. pneumoniae, 20 percent to L. monocytogenes, and 3 to 4 percent each to N. meningitidis, group B streptococcus, and H. influenzae. An increased prevalence of L. monocytogenes occurs in the elderly.
   B. **Predisposing factors.** Major mechanisms for developing meningitis:
      1. Colonization of the nasopharynx with subsequent bloodstream invasion and subsequent central nervous system (CNS) invasion
      2. Invasion of the CNS following bacteremia due to a localized source, such as infective endocarditis or a urinary tract infection
      3. Direct entry of organisms into the CNS from a contiguous infection (eg, sinuses, mastoid), trauma, neurosurgery, or medical devices (eg, shunts or intracerebral pressure monitors).
   C. Host factors that can predispose to meningitis include asplenia, complement deficiency, corticosteroid excess, and HIV infection. Other predisposing factors for meningitis include:
      1. Recent exposure to someone with meningitis
      2. A recent infection (especially respiratory or otic infection)
      3. Recent travel, particularly to areas with endemic meningococcal disease such as sub-Saharan Africa
      4. Injection drug use
      5. Recent head trauma
      6. Otorrhea or rhinorrhea
II. **Clinical features.** Patients with bacterial meningitis appear ill and often present soon after symptom onset.
   A. **Presenting manifestations.** The classic triad of acute bacterial meningitis consists of fever, nuchal rigidity, and a change in mental status, although many patients do not have all three features. Most patients have high fevers, often greater than 38°C, but a small percentage have hypothermia.
   B. Headache is also common. The headache is severe and generalized. It is not easily confused with normal headaches.
   C. Fever is present in 95 percent at presentation and developed in another 4 percent within the first 24 hours.

D. Nuchal rigidity is present in 88 percent.

E. Mental status is altered in 78 percent. Most were confused or lethargic, but 22 percent are responsive only to pain and 6 percent are unresponsive to all stimuli.

F. Significant photophobia is common.

G. Neurologic complications such as seizures, focal neurologic deficits (including cranial nerve palsies), and papilledema, may be present early or occur later in the course. Seizures occur in 15 to 30 percent and focal neurologic deficits in 20 to 30 percent. Hearing loss is a late complication. Dexamethasone therapy may reduce the rate of neurologic sequelae.

H. N. meningitidis can cause petechiae and palpable purpura.

I. **Examination for nuchal rigidity.** Passive or active flexion of the neck will usually result in an inability to touch the chin to the chest.

    1. Brudzinski sign refers to spontaneous flexion of the hips during flexion of the neck.

    2. The Kernig sign refers to the inability or reluctance to allow full extension of the knee when the hip is flexed 90°.

    3. The sensitivity of meningeal signs is extremely low (5 percent for each sign and 30 percent for nuchal rigidity); the specificity was 95 percent for each sign and 68 percent for nuchal rigidity.

J. **Initial blood tests** should include a complete blood count with differential and platelet count, and two sets of blood cultures. A specimen of cerebrospinal fluid (CSF) should be obtained for cell count and differential, glucose and protein concentration, Gram stain, and culture. Characteristic findings in bacterial meningitis include a CSF glucose concentration below 45 mg/dL, a protein concentration above 500 mg/dL, and a white blood cell count above 1000/microL, usually composed primarily of neutrophils. Most often the white blood cell count is elevated with a shift toward immature forms. Severe infection can be associated with leukopenia. The platelet count may be reduced if disseminated intravascular coagulation or meningococcal bacteremia is present.

    1. **Blood cultures** are often positive. Approximately 50 to 75 percent of patients with bacterial meningitis have positive blood cultures. Cultures obtained after antimicrobial therapy are much less likely to be positive, particularly for meningococcus. Tests of serum and urine for bacterial antigens are unhelpful.

K. **Lumbar puncture.** Every patient with suspected meningitis should have CSF obtained unless the procedure is contraindicated. Risk factors for an occult mass lesion on CT scan include the presence of impaired cellular immunity, history of previous central nervous system disease, a seizure within the previous week, reduced level of consciousness, and focal motor or cranial abnormalities. A CT scan is recommended before an LP only in patients with suspected bacterial meningitis who have one or more risk factors for a mass lesion.

    1. **Opening pressure** is typically elevated in patients with bacterial meningitis. The mean opening pressure is 350 mm H_2O (normal up to 200 mm H_2O).

    2. **CSF analysis.** When the clinical diagnosis strongly suggests meningitis, CSF Gram stain, culture, and analysis can distinguish between bacterial and viral infection. A Gram stain should be obtained whenever there is suspicion of bacterial meningitis. The following findings may be seen:

    3. Gram positive diplococci suggest pneumococcal infection.

    4. Gram negative diplococci suggest meningococcal infection.

5. Small pleomorphic Gram negative coccobacilli suggest Haemophilus influenzae.
6. Gram positive rods and coccobacilli suggest listerial infection.

Utility of CSF Analysis in Infectious Causes of CNS Infection

	Glucose		Protein		Total WBC		
	<10 mg/dL	10-45 mg/dL	>500 mg/dL	50-500 mg/dL	>1000	100-1000	5-100
More common	Bacterial meningitis	Bacterial meningitis	Bacterial meningitis	Viral meningitis	Bacterial meningitis	Bacterial or viral meningitis	Early bacterial meningitis
				Lyme disease			Viral meningitis
				Meningeal syphilis			Meningeal syphilis
							TB meningitis
Less common	TB meningitis	Meningeal syphilis	TB meningitis		Some cases of mumps	Encephalitis (including West Nile virus)	Encephalitis (including Herpes simplex virus)

Common self-limited forms of viral meningitis usually have a CSF protein concentration below 100 mg/dL (1 g/L) and a total WBC less than 100/μL. In addition to the total WBC, the percent neutrophils also may be helpful: more than 50 percent suggests bacterial meningitis while a value below 10 percent is compatible with viral infection

III. Treatment of bacterial meningitis in adults

A. Antibiotic therapy should be initiated immediately after the results of lumbar puncture (LP) or immediately after LP alone if the clinical suspicion is high. A screening CT scan is not necessary in the majority of patients. Risk factors for cerebral herniation include presence of impaired cellular immunity, history of previous central nervous system disease, or a seizure within the previous week reduced level of consciousness, focal motor or cranial abnormalities, and papilledema. Should LP be delayed by the need for cranial imaging, blood cultures should be obtained and antibiotics should be administered empirically before the imaging study, followed as

soon as possible by the LP. In addition, dexamethasone (0.15 mg/kg IV every six hours) should be given shortly before or at the same time as the antibiotics clinical and laboratory evidence suggests bacterial meningitis.
- B. **Empiric drug regimen.** Selected third-generation cephalosporins, such as cefotaxime and ceftriaxone, are the beta-lactams of choice in the empiric treatment of meningitis.
    1. Cefotaxime and ceftriaxone are equivalent or superior to penicillin and ampicillin because of their consistent CSF penetration and their activity against the major pathogens of meningitis with one notable exception, some penicillin-resistant S. pneumoniae. Ceftazidime, another third-generation cephalosporin, is much less active against penicillin-resistant pneumococci than cefotaxime and ceftriaxone.

Empiric antibiotic therapy in adults with suspected bacterial meningitis and a nondiagnostic CSF gram stain

Suggested antibiotics	Most likely pathogens
Immunocompetent adults	
Age 18 to 60 years Ceftriaxone (2 g twice daily) **OR,** less preferably, cefotaxime (2 g every four to six or six to eight hours) **AND** vancomycin (2 g/day in two to four divided doses) if cephalosporin-resistant pneumococci in community	S. Pneumoniae, N. Meningitis H. influenzae, and, much less often, L. monocytogenes and group B streptococci
Age ≥60 years As above plus ampicillin (200 mg/kg per day in six divided doses)	S. Pneumoniae, L. monocytogenes, and, less often, group B streptococci, N. Meningitis, H. influenzae
Impaired cellular immunity Ceftazidime (2 g every eight hours) **PLUS** Ampicillin (2 g every four hours) **AND** vancomycin (2 g/day in two to four divided doses) if cephalosporin-resistant pneumococci in community	L. Monocytogenes, gram negative bacilli

    2. Intravenous antibiotics should be directed at the presumed pathogen if the Gram stain is diagnostic. Antibiotic therapy should then be modified once the CSF culture results are available.
        a. If Gram positive cocci are seen in community-acquired meningitis, S. pneumoniae should be the suspected pathogen. However, in the setting of neurosurgery or head trauma within the past month, a neurosurgical device, or a CSF leak, Staphylococcus aureus and

coagulase negative staphylococci are more common and vancomycin is required.

b. If Gram negative cocci are seen, N. meningitidis is the probable pathogen.

c. Gram positive bacilli suggest Listeria.

d. Gram negative bacilli usually represent Enterobacteriaceae (eg, Klebsiella, Escherichia coli) in cases of community-acquired meningitis.

e. If there is a history of neurosurgery or head trauma within the past month, a neurosurgical device, or a CSF leak in patients with Gram negative rods, ceftriaxone should be replaced with ceftazidime since such patients are at greater risk for Pseudomonas and Acinetobacter infection.

C. **Adjuvant dexamethasone.** Permanent neurologic sequelae, such as hearing loss and focal neurologic deficits, are not uncommon in survivors of bacterial meningitis, particularly with pneumococcal meningitis. Intravenous dexamethasone (0.15 mg/kg every six hours) should be given shortly before or at the time of initiation of antibiotic therapy in adults with suspected bacterial meningitis who have a Glasgow coma score of 8 to 11. Dexamethasone should be continued for four days if the Gram stain or the CSF culture reveals S. pneumoniae. Dexamethasone should be discontinued if the Gram stain and/or culture reveal another pathogen or no meningitis.

D. **Choice of agent when pathogen is unknown.** Antibiotic selection must be empiric when lumbar puncture is delayed or Gram stain of the CSF does not reveal a pathogen.

1. In adults up to age 60, S. pneumoniae was responsible for 60 percent of cases, followed by N. meningitidis (20 percent), H. influenzae (10 percent), L. monocytogenes (6 percent), and group B streptococcus (4 percent).

2. In adults $\geq$60 years of age, almost 70 percent of cases are caused by S. pneumoniae, 20 percent to L. monocytogenes, and 3 to 4 percent each to N. meningitidis, group B streptococcus, and H. influenzae. An increased prevalence of L. monocytogenes in the elderly has been noted.

3. **No known immune deficiency.** Meningococcus, pneumococcus, and, less often, H. influenzae and group B streptococcus are the most likely causes of community-acquired bacterial meningitis in adolescents and adults up to the age of 60. Such patients should be treated with intravenous ceftriaxone (2 g BID) or cefotaxime (2 g every six to eight hours). If cephalosporin resistance occurs in more than 3 percent S. pneumoniae isolates, vancomycin should be added (2 g/day intravenously in two to four divided doses if renal function is normal). Beta-lactams should be continued even if in vitro tests suggest possible intermediate or resistant organisms, since they will provide synergy with vancomycin. Adults $\geq$60 years of age, in whom 20 percent of cases are due to listeria, should receive ampicillin (200 mg/kg per day IV in six divided doses).

Antibiotic recommendations for adults with suspected meningitis with a positive cerebrospinal fluid gram stain or culture	
Bacterial type	**Recommended antibiotic regimen**
Morphology on CSF Gram stain	
Gram positive cocci	Vancomycin (500 mg Q6h)‡ **PLUS** either ceftriaxone (2 g Q12h) or, less preferably, cefotaxime (2 g Q4-6h or Q6-8h)
Gram negative cocci	Penicillin G (4 million U Q4h) or, if H. Influenzae (which typically appears as small, pleomorphic rods) is suspected, ceftriaxone (2 g Q12h) or cefotaxime (2 g Q6-8h)
Gram positive bacilli	Ampicillin (2 g Q4h) **PLUS** gentamicin (1-2 mg/kg Q8h)
Gram negative bacilli	Ceftriaxone (2 g Q12h) or cefotaxime (2 g Q6-8h) **PLUS** gentamicin (1-2 mg/kg Q8h)
Growth in CSF culture	
S. pneumoniae	Vancomycin (500 mg Q6h)‡ **PLUS** either ceftriaxone (2 g Q12h) or, less preferably, cefotaxime (2 g Q4-6h or Q6-8h) for 14 days; vancomycin can be discontinued if the isolate is not cephalosporin-resistant
N. meningitis	Penicillin G (4 million units Q4h) for seven days
H. influenzae	Ceftriaxone (2 g Q12h) or cefotaxime (2 g Q6h) for seven days
L. Monocytogenes	Ampicillin (2 g Q4h) or penicillin G (3-4 million U Q4h) **PLUS** gentamicin (1-2 mg/kg Q8h); ampicillin is given for two to four weeks in immunocompetent patients and for at lease six to eight weeks in immunocompromised patients; gentamicin is gen until the patient improves (usually 10 to 14 days) or, in poor responders, for up to three weeks if there are no signs of nephrotoxicity and ototoxicity
Group B streptococci	Penicillin G (4 million U Q4h) for two to three weeks

Bacterial type	Recommended antibiotic regimen
Enterobacteriaceae	Ceftriaxone (2 g Q12h) or cefotaxime (2 g Q6h-8h) **PLUS** gentamicin (1-2 mg/kg Q8h) for three weeks
Pseudomonas or acinetobacter	ceftazidime (2 g Q8h) **PLUS** gentamicin (1-2 mg/kg Q8h) for 21 days

4. **Impaired cellular immunity** due to lymphoma, cytotoxic chemotherapy, or high-dose glucocorticoids requires coverage against L. monocytogenes and Gram negative bacilli as well as S. pneumoniae. Patients should receive ceftazidime (2 g every eight hours) and ampicillin (200 mg/kg per day IV in six divided doses). Vancomycin should be added (2 g/day intravenously in two to four divided doses if renal function is normal) if there is possible cephalosporin-resistant pneumococci.

5. **Nosocomial infection.** Empiric therapy must cover both Gram negative (such as Klebsiella pneumoniae and Pseudomonas aeruginosa) and Gram positive nosocomial pathogens. Ceftazidime (2 g every eight hours) plus vancomycin (2 g/day intravenously in two to four divided doses if renal function is normal) is recommended.

E. Prevention
  1. **Vaccines** are available for S. pneumoniae, N. meningitidis, and H. influenzae.
    a. **Pneumococcal vaccine** is administered to chronically ill and older adults (over age 65).
    b. **Meningococcal vaccine** is not warranted as postexposure prophylaxis unless the strain is documented to have a capsular serotype represented in the vaccine (type A, C, Y or W-135). Meningococcal vaccination is indicated for patients with asplenia and complement deficiencies.
    c. **H. influenzae vaccine.** A marked reduction in H. influenzae meningitis has been associated with the near universal use of a H. influenzae vaccine.
  2. **Chemoprophylaxis**
    a. **Neisseria meningitidis.** Chemoprophylaxis of close contacts consists of rifampin (600 mg PO every 12 h for a total of four doses in adults), ciprofloxacin (500 mg PO once), and ceftriaxone (250 mg IM once).

Antimicrobial chemoprophylaxis regimens for meningococcal infection			
Drug	**Age group**	**Dose**	**Duration**
Rifampin (oral)	Children <1 month	5 mg/kg every 12 hours	Two days
	Children >1 month	20 mg/kg every 12 hours	Two days
	Adults	600 mg every 12 hours	Two days
Ciprofloxacin (IM)	Adults	500 mg	Single dose
Ceftriaxone (IM)	Children ≤12 years	125 mg	Single dose
	Older children and adults	250 mg	Single dose

   b. **H. influenzae.** Unvaccinated, young children (less than four years of
      age) who have close contact with patients with H. influenzae type b
      meningitis require rifampin (20 mg/kg with a max of 600 mg/day PO
      for four days).

Community-Acquired Pneumonia

Four million cases of Community-acquired pneumonia (CAP) occur annually.
Bacteria are the most common cause of pneumonia and have been divided into
two groups: "typical" and "atypical": "Typical" organisms include Streptococcus
pneumoniae, Haemophilus influenzae, Staphylococcus aureus, and other Gram
negative bacteria. Atypical" refers to pneumonia caused by Legionella sp,
Mycoplasma pneumoniae, and Chlamydia pneumoniae.

I. Pathophysiology
A. Pneumococcal pneumonia
   1. S. pneumoniae is the most common cause of CAP. The organism is
      isolated in only 5 to 18 percent. Risk factors for pneumococcal
      pneumonia include: advanced age, cigarette smoking, dementia,
      malnutrition, the presence of chronic illnesses, and human immunodefi-
      ciency virus (HIV) infection.
   2. Pneumonia caused by pneumococcus is usually associated with
      cough, sputum production, and fever. Bacteremia accompanies the
      pneumonia in 20 to 30 percent of cases. A parapneumonic pleural
      effusion is present in the majority of patients, but empyema occurs in
      only two percent of cases.
   3. Penicillin resistance is an increasing problem.
B. Other bacteria. H. influenzae (generally other than type B), S. aureus,
      Legionella, and Gram negative bacteria each account for 3 to 10 percent
      of cases of CAP.

1. The patient population and clinical presentation of H. influenzae pneumonia is similar to that with pneumococcal disease.
2. S. aureus pneumonia that is community-acquired is usually seen in the elderly and in younger patients who are recovering from influenza (post-influenza pneumonia).
3. Legionella accounts for 2 to 8 percent of cases of CAP. Among patients with pneumonia who can be treated as outpatients, the frequency of Legionnaires' disease is less than 1 percent. Legionella is much more frequent in hospitalized patients, especially those admitted to intensive care units.
4. Gram-negative bacilli, especially P. aeruginosa, are an uncommon cause of CAP except in patients with neutropenia, cystic fibrosis, late stage HIV infection and bronchiectasis.
5. Other bacteria that can cause CAP include Neisseria meningitidis, Moraxella catarrhalis, and Streptococcus pyogenes.
6. Anaerobic organisms may be the cause of aspiration pneumonia and lung abscess.

II. Diagnostic approach

A. **Clinical evaluation.** CAP caused by pyogenic organisms presents with the sudden onset of rigors, fever, pleuritic chest pain, and cough productive of purulent sputum. Chest pain occurs in 30 percent of cases, chills in 40 to 50 percent, and rigors in 15 percent.

B. On physical examination, 80 percent are febrile, although this finding is frequently absent in older patients. A respiratory rate above 24 breaths/minute is noted in 45 to 70 percent of patients; tachycardia is also common. Chest examination reveals audible rales in most patients, while one-third have consolidation.

C. The major blood test abnormality is leukocytosis (15,000 and 30,000 per mm^3) with a leftward shift. Leukopenia can occur.

D. **Chest radiographs.** The presence of an infiltrate on plain chest radiograph is the "gold standard" for diagnosing pneumonia. The radiographic appearances include lobar consolidation, interstitial infiltrates, and cavitation.

E. **Sputum examination.** An etiologic agent is found in 51 percent of patients. A specimen that has greater than 25 PMN and less than 10 epithelial cells per low power field represents a purulent specimen. Gram stain and culture may identify the cause of the pneumonia.

F. **Blood cultures** should be obtained in patients who require hospitalization.

G. **Urinary antigen testing** for pneumococcal cell wall components has a sensitivity of 70 to 90 percent; specificity is 80 to 100 percent. Urinary antigen testing is also available for Legionella species and is highly sensitive and specific and inexpensive. Urinary antigen testing is recommended for both S. pneumoniae and Legionella, particularly in patients with risk factors for Legionella infection (eg, smoking, chronic lung disease, immunosuppression, and CAP requiring hospitalization).

Causes of Community-acquired Pneumonia	
Etiology	**Prevalence (percent)**
Streptococcus pneumoniae	20-60
Hemophilus influenzae	3-10
Staphylococcus aureus	3-5
Gram-negative bacilli	3-10
Aspiration	6-10
Miscellaneous	3-5
Legionella sp.	2-8
Mycoplasma pneumoniae	1-6
Chlamydia pneumoniae	4-6
Viruses	2-15

III. Treatment of Community-Acquired Pneumonia

A. Empiric regimens. For uncomplicated pneumonia in patients who do not require hospitalization, macrolide therapy is recommended. Erythromycin is the least expensive macrolide but is associated with gastrointestinal upset in many patients. Azithromycin (Zithromax [500 mg PO QD]) is recommended because it causes less gastrointestinal upset; if macrolide resistance in the community is high, doxycycline (100 mg PO twice a day) should be considered. Telithromycin (Ketek) or a quinolone is also reasonable if macrolide resistance is prevalent. Quinolones are not recommended for patients with CAP because achievable tissue concentrations of these agents will be close to the minimum inhibitory concentration for pneumococcus and resistance may emerge with overuse.

B. Duration of therapy. The usual recommended duration of therapy is 7 to 14 days. Three days of azithromycin may be as effective as longer course of antibiotics. For a hospitalized patient, ceftriaxone (Rocephin [2 g IV QD]) with or without azithromycin (depending upon the likelihood of an atypical organism) is recommended. For more severely ill patients who might have an atypical pneumonia or patients admitted to an ICU, therapy consists of a quinolone, such as levofloxacin (Levaquin [500 mg IV QD]) or azithromycin to treat legionella infection as well as mycoplasma and chlamydia. Consideration should be given to adding a second agent for pneumococcus to levofloxacin. Ceftriaxone should be given with azithromycin in these sicker patients.

Recommended Empiric Drug Therapy for Patients with Community-Acquired Pneumonia		
Clinical Situation	**Primary Treatment**	**Alternative(s)**
Younger (<60 yr) out-patients without un-derlying disease	Macrolide antibiotics (azithromycin, clarithromycin, dirithromycin, or erythromycin)	Levofloxacin or doxycycline

Clinical Situation	Primary Treatment	Alternative(s)
Older (>60 yr) outpatients with underlying disease	Levofloxacin or cefuroxime or Trimethoprim-sulfamethoxazole Add vancomycin in severe, life-threatening pneumonias	Beta-lactamase inhibitor (with macrolide if legionella infection suspected)
Gross aspiration suspected	Clindamycin IV	Cefotetan, ampicillin/sulbactam

Common Antimicrobial Agents for Community-Acquired Pneumonia in Adults

Type	Agent	Dosage
Oral therapy		
Macrolides	Erythromycin Clarithromycin (Biaxin) Azithromycin (Zithromax)	500 mg PO qid 500 mg PO bid 500 mg PO on day 1, then 250 mg qd x 4 days
Beta-lactam/beta-lactamase inhibitor	Amoxicillin-clavulanate (Augmentin) Augmentin XR	500 mg tid or 875 mg PO bid 2 tabs q12h
Quinolones	Ciprofloxacin (Cipro) Levofloxacin (Levaquin) Ofloxacin (Floxin)	500 mg PO bid 500 mg PO qd 400 mg PO bid
Tetracycline	Doxycycline	100 m g PO bid
Sulfonamide	Trimethoprim-sulfamethoxazole	160 mg/800 mg (DS) PO bid
Intravenous Therapy		
Cephalosporins Second-generation Third-generation (anti-Pseudomonas aeruginosa)	Cefuroxime (Kefurox, Zinacef) Ceftizoxime (Cefizox) Ceftazidime (Fortaz) Cefoperazone (Cefobid)	0.75-1.5 g IV q8h 1-2 g IV q8h 1-2 g IV q8h 1-2 g IV q8h
Beta-lactam/beta-lactamase inhibitors	Ampicillin-sulbactam (Unasyn) Piperacillin/tazobactam (Zosyn) Ticarcillin-clavulanate (Timentin)	1.5 g IV q6h 3.375 g IV q6h 3.1 g IV q6h

Type	Agent	Dosage
Quinolones	Ciprofloxacin (Cipro) Levofloxacin (Levaquin) Ofloxacin (Floxin)	400 mg IV q12h 500 mg IV q24h 400 mg IV q12h
Aminoglycosides	Gentamicin Amikacin	Load 2.0 mg/kg IV, then 1.5 mg/kg q8h
Vancomycin	Vancomycin	1 gm IV q12h

A. Patients initially treated with intravenous antibiotics can be switched to oral agents when the patient is afebrile. The regimens for the hospitalized patient are also appropriate for patients admitted from long-term care facilities. Discharged from the hospital may be completed once oral therapy.

B. Most patients respond to a course of 10 to 14 days of antibiotics, although 3 to 5 days of azithromycin is an alternative in ambulatory patients.

C. **Response to therapy.** Some improvement in the patient's clinical course should be seen within 48 to 72 hours. Fever in patients with lobar pneumonia often takes 72 hours or longer to improve. The chest x-ray usually clears within four weeks in patients younger than 50 years of age without underlying pulmonary disease.

D. The nonresponding patient
  1. If the patient does not improve within 72 hours, an organism which is not covered by the initial antibiotic regimen should be considered. This could be the result of drug resistance, nonbacterial infection, unusual pathogens (eg, Pneumocystis carinii or Mycobacterium tuberculosis), drug fever, or a complication such as postobstructive pneumonia, empyema, or abscess. The differential diagnosis also includes noninfectious etiologies, such as malignancy, inflammatory conditions, or heart failure.
  2. When evaluating a patient who is not responding to therapy, it is important to repeat the history to include travel and pet exposures to look for unusual pathogens. Bronchoscopy can be performed to evaluate the airway for obstruction due to a foreign body or malignancy. Previously unsuspected pathogens may include P. carinii or M. tuberculosis.

Pneumocystis Carinii Pneumonia

PCP is the most common life-threatening opportunistic infection occurring in patients with HIV disease. In the era of PCP prophylaxis and highly active antiretroviral therapy, the incidence of PCP is decreasing. The incidence of PCP has declined steadily from 50% in 1987 to 25% currently.

I. **Risk factors for Pneumocystis carinii pneumonia**
  A. Patients with CD4 counts of 200 cells/µL or less are 4.9 times more likely to develop PCP.
  B. Candidates for PCP prophylaxis include: patients with a prior history of PCP, patients with a CD4 cell count of less than 200 cells/µL, and HIV-infected patients with thrush or persistent fever.

II. Clinical presentation

A. PCP usually presents with fever, dry cough, and shortness of breath or dyspnea on exertion with a gradual onset over several weeks. Tachypnea may be pronounced. Circumoral, acral, and mucous membrane cyanosis may be evident.

B. Laboratory findings

  1. Complete blood count and sedimentation rate shows no characteristic pattern in patients with PCP. The serum LDH concentration is frequently increased.

  2. Arterial blood gas measurements generally show increases in P(A-a)O_2, although PaO_2 values vary widely depending on disease severity. Up to 25% of patients may have a PaO_2 of 80 mm Hg or above while breathing room air.

  3. Pulmonary function tests. Patients with PCP usually have a decreased diffusing capacity for carbon monoxide (DLCO).

C. Radiographic presentation

  1. PCP in AIDS patients usually causes a diffuse interstitial infiltrate. High resolution computerized tomography (HRCT) may be helpful for those patients who have normal chest radiographic findings.

  2. Pneumatoceles (cavities, cysts, blebs, or bullae) and spontaneous pneumothoraces are common in patients with PCP.

III. Laboratory diagnosis

A. Sputum induction. The least invasive means of establishing a specific diagnosis is the examination of sputum induced by inhalation of a 3-5% saline mist. The sensitivity of induced sputum examination for PCP is 74-77% and the negative predictive value is 58-64%. If the sputum tests negative, an invasive diagnostic procedure is required to confirm the diagnosis of PCP.

B. Transbronchial biopsy and bronchoalveolar lavage. The sensitivity of transbronchial biopsy for PCP is 98%. The sensitivity of bronchoalveolar is 90%.

C. Open-lung biopsy should be reserved for patients with progressive pulmonary disease in whom the less invasive procedures are nondiagnostic.

IV. Diagnostic algorithm

A. If the chest radiograph of a symptomatic patient appears normal, a DLCO should be performed. Patients with significant symptoms, a normal-appearing chest radiograph, and a normal DLCO should undergo high-resolution CT. Patients with abnormal findings at any of these steps should proceed to sputum induction or bronchoscopy. Sputum specimens collected by induction that reveal P. carinii should also be stained for acid-fast organisms and fungi, and the specimen should be cultured for mycobacteria and fungi.

B. Patients whose sputum examinations do not show P. carinii or another pathogen should undergo bronchoscopy.

C. Lavage fluid is stained for P. carinii, acid-fast organisms, and fungi. Also, lavage fluid is cultured for mycobacteria and fungi and inoculated onto cell culture for viral isolation. Touch imprints are made from tissue specimens and stained for P. carinii. Fluid is cultured for mycobacteria and fungi, and stained for P. carinii, acid-fast organisms, and fungi. If all procedures are nondiagnostic and the lung disease is progressive, open-lung biopsy may be considered.

V. Treatment of Pneumocystic carinii pneumonia

A. **Trimethoprim-sulfamethoxazole DS (Bactrim DS, Septra DS)** is the recommended initial therapy for PCP. Dosage is 15-20 mg/kg/day of TMP IV divided q6h for 14-21 days. Adverse effects include rash (33%), elevation of liver enzymes (44%), nausea and vomiting (50%), anemia (40%), creatinine elevation (33%), and hyponatremia (94%).

B. **Pentamidine** is an alternative in patients who have adverse reactions or fail to respond to TMP-SMX. The dosage is 4 mg/kg/day IV for 14-21 days. Adverse effects include anemia (33%), creatinine elevation (60%), LFT elevation (63%), and hyponatremia (56%). Pancreatitis, hypoglycemia, and hyperglycemia are common side effects.

C. **Corticosteroids.** Adjunctive corticosteroid treatment is beneficial with anti-PCP therapy in patients with a partial pressure of oxygen (PaO_2) less than 70 mm Hg, (A-a)DO_2 greater than 35 mm Hg, or oxygen saturation less than 90% on room air. Contraindications include suspected tuberculosis or disseminated fungal infection. Treatment with methylprednisolone (SoluMedrol) should begin at the same time as anti-PCP therapy. The dosage is 30 mg IV q12h x 5 days, then 30 mg IV qd x 5 days, then 15 mg qd x 11 days **OR** prednisone, 40 mg twice daily for 5 days, then 40 mg daily for 5 days, and then 20 mg daily until day 21 of therapy.

VI. Prophylaxis

A. HIV-infected patients who have CD4 counts less than 200 cells/mcL should receive prophylaxis against PCP. If CD4 count increases to greater than 200 cells/mcL after receiving antiretroviral therapy, PCP prophylaxis can be safely discontinued.

B. **Trimethoprim-sulfamethoxazole** (once daily to three times weekly) is the preferred regimen for PCP prophylaxis.

C. **Dapsone** (100 mg daily or twice weekly) is a prophylactic regimen for patients who can not tolerate TMP-SMX.

D. **Aerosolized pentamidine (NebuPent)** 300 mg in 6 mL water nebulized over x 20 min q4 weeks is another alternative.

Antiretroviral Therapy and Opportunistic Infections in AIDS

I. Antiretroviral therapy

A. A combination of three agents is recommended as initial therapy. The preferred options are 2 nucleosides plus 1 protease inhibitor or 1 non-nucleoside. Alternative options are 2 protease inhibitors plus 1 nucleoside or 1 non-nucleoside. Combinations of 1 nucleoside, 1 non-nucleoside, and 1 protease inhibitor are also effective.

B. **Nucleoside analogs**
1. Abacavir (Ziagen) 300 mg PO bid [300 mg].
2. Didanosine (Videx) 200 mg PO bid [chewable tabs: 25, 50, 100, 150 mg]; oral ulcers discourage common usage.
3. Lamivudine (Epivir) 150 mg PO bid [tab: 150 mg].
4. Stavudine (Zerit) 40 mg PO bid [cap: 15, 20, 30, 40 mg].
5. Zalcitabine (Hivid) 0.75 mg PO tid [tab: 0.375, 0.75 mg].
6. Zidovudine (Retrovir, AZT) 200 mg PO tid or 300 mg PO bid [cap: 100, 300 mg].
7. Zidovudine 300 mg/lamivudine 150 mg (Combivir) 1 tab PO bid.

    C. Protease inhibitors
        1. Amprenavir (Agenerase) 1200 mg PO bid [50, 150 mg]
        2. Indinavir (Crixivan) 800 mg PO tid [cap: 200, 400 mg].
        3. Nelfinavir (Viracept) 750 mg PO tid [tab: 250 mg]
        4. Ritonavir (Norvir) 600 mg PO bid [cap: 100 mg].
        5. Saquinavir (Invirase) 600 mg PO tid [cap: 200 mg].
    D. Non-nucleoside analogs
        1. Delavirdine (Rescriptor) 400 mg PO tid [tab: 100 mg]
        2. Efavirenz (Sustiva) 600 mg qhs [50, 100, 200 mg]
        3. Nevirapine (Viramune) 200 mg PO bid [tab: 200 mg]

II. Oral candidiasis
    A. Fluconazole (Diflucan), acute: 200 mg PO x 1, then 100 mg qd x 5 days
    OR
    B. Ketoconazole (Nizoral), acute: 400 mg po qd 1-2 weeks or until resolved
    OR
    C. Clotrimazole (Mycelex) troches 10 mg dissolved slowly in mouth 5 times/d.

III.   **Candida esophagitis**
    A. Fluconazole (Diflucan) 200 mg PO x 1, then 100 mg PO qd until improved.
    B. Ketoconazole (Nizoral) 200 mg po bid.

IV.   **Primary or recurrent mucocutaneous HSV**. Acyclovir (Zovirax), 200-400 mg PO 5 times a day for 10 days, or 5 mg/kg IV q8h; or in cases of acyclovir resistance, foscarnet 40 mg/kg IV q8h for 21 days.

V. Herpes simplex encephalitis. Acyclovir 10 mg/kg IV q8h x 10-21 days.

VI.   **Herpes varicella zoster**
    A. Acyclovir (Zovirax) 10 mg/kg IV over 60 min q8h **OR**
    B. Valacyclovir (Valtrex) 1000 mg PO tid x 7 days [caplet: 500 mg].

VII. Cytomegalovirus infections
    A. Ganciclovir (Cytovene) 5 mg/kg IV (dilute in 100 mL D5W over 60 min) q12h x 14-21 days (concurrent use with zidovudine increases hematological toxicity).
    B. Suppressive treatment for CMV: Ganciclovir (Cytovene) 5 mg/kg IV qd, or 6 mg/kg IV 5 times/wk, or 1000 mg orally tid with food.

VIII. **Toxoplasmosis**
    A. Pyrimethamine 200 mg PO loading dose, then 50-75 mg qd plus leucovorin calcium (folinic acid) 10-20 mg PO qd for 6-8 weeks for acute therapy **AND**
    B. Sulfadiazine (1.0-1.5 gm PO q6h) or clindamycin 450 mg PO qid/600-900 mg IV q6h.
    C. Suppressive treatment for toxoplasmosis
        1. Pyrimethamine 25-50 mg PO qd with or without sulfadiazine 0.5-1.0 gm PO q6h; and folinic acid 5-10 mg PO qd **OR**
        2. Pyrimethamine 50 mg PO qd; and clindamycin 300 mg PO q6h; and folinic acid 5-10 mg PO qd.

IX. Cryptococcus neoformans meningitis
    A. Amphotericin B at 0.7 mg/kg/d IV for 14 days or until clinically stable, followed by fluconazole (Diflucan) 400 mg qd to complete 10 weeks of therapy, followed by suppressive therapy with fluconazole (Diflucan) 200 mg PO qd indefinitely.
    B. Amphotericin B lipid complex (Abelcet) may be used in place of non-liposomal amphotericin B if the patient is intolerant to non-liposomal amphotericin B. The dosage is 5 mg/kg IV q24h.

X. Active tuberculosis
  A. Isoniazid (INH) 300 mg PO qd; and rifabutin 300 mg PO qd; and pyrazinamide 15-25 mg/kg PO qd (500 mg PO bid-tid); and ethambutol 15-25 mg/kg PO qd (400 mg PO bid-tid).
  B. All four drugs are continued for 2 months; isoniazid and rifabutin (depending on susceptibility testing) are continued for a period of at least 9 months and at least 6 months after the last negative cultures.
  C. Pyridoxine (vitamin B6) 50 mg PO qd, concurrent with INH.

XI. Disseminated mycobacterium avium complex (MAC)
  A. Azithromycin (Zithromax) 500-1000 mg PO qd or clarithromycin (Biaxin) 500 mg PO bid; **AND**
  B. Ethambutol 15-25 mg/kg PO qd (400 mg bid-tid) **AND**
  C. Rifabutin 300 mg/d (two 150 mg tablets qd).
  D. Prophylaxis for MAC
   1. Clarithromycin (Biaxin) 500 mg PO bid **OR**
   2. Rifabutin (Mycobutin) 300 mg PO qd or 150 mg PO bid.

XII. Disseminated coccidioidomycosis
  A. Amphotericin B (Fungizone) 0.8 mg/kg IV qd **OR**
  B. Amphotericin B lipid complex (Abelcet) 5 mg/kg IV q24h **OR**
  C. Fluconazole (Diflucan) 400-800 mg PO or IV qd.

XIII. Disseminated histoplasmosis
  A. Amphotericin B (Fungizone) 0.5-0.8 mg/kg IV qd, until total dose 15 mg/kg **OR**
  B. Amphotericin B lipid complex (Abelcet) 5 mg/kg IV q24h **OR**
  C. Itraconazole (Sporanox) 200 mg PO bid.
  D. **Suppressive treatment for histoplasmosis:** Itraconazole (Sporanox) 200 mg PO bid.

Sepsis

About 400,000 cases of sepsis, 200,000 cases of septic shock, and 100,000 deaths from both occur each year.

I. Pathophysiology
  A. Sepsis is defined as the systemic response to infection. In the absence of infection, it is called systemic inflammatory response syndrome and is characterized by at least two of the following: temperature greater than 38°C or less than 36°C; heart rate greater than 90 beats per minute; respiratory rate more than 20/minute or $PaCO_2$ less than 32 mm Hg; and an alteration in white blood cell count (>12,000/mm³ or <4,000/mm³).
  B. Septic shock is defined as sepsis-induced hypotension that persists despite fluid resuscitation and is associated with tissue hypoperfusion.
  C. The initial cardiovascular response to sepsis includes decreased systemic vascular resistance and depressed ventricular function. Low systemic vascular resistance occurs. If this initial cardiovascular response is uncompensated, generalized tissue hypoperfusion results. Aggressive fluid resuscitation may improve cardiac output and systemic blood pressure, resulting in the typical hemodynamic pattern of septic shock (ie, high cardiac index and low systemic vascular resistance).
  D. Although gram-negative bacteremia is commonly found in patients with sepsis, gram-positive infection may affect 30-40% of patients. Fungal, viral

and parasitic infections are usually encountered in immunocompromised patients.

Defining sepsis and related disorders	
Term	**Definition**
Systemic inflammatory response syndrome (SIRS)	The systemic inflammatory response to a severe clinical insult manifested by >2 of the following conditions: Temperature >38°C or <36°C, heart rate >90 beats/min, respiratory rate >20 breaths/min or $PaCO_2$ <32 mm Hg, white blood cell count >12,000 cells/mm^3 , <4000 cells/mm^3 , or >10% band cells
Sepsis	The presence of SIRS caused by an infectious process; sepsis is considered severe if hypotension or systemic manifestations of hypoperfusion (lactic acidosis, oliguria, change in mental status) is present.
Septic shock	Sepsis-induced hypotension despite adequate fluid resuscitation, along with the presence of perfusion abnormalities that may induce lactic acidosis, oliguria, or an alteration in mental status.
Multiple organ dysfunction syndrome (MODS)	The presence of altered organ function in an acutely ill patient such that homeostasis cannot be maintained without intervention

- **E.** Sources of bacteremia leading to sepsis include the urinary, respiratory and GI tracts, and skin and soft tissues (including catheter sites). The source of bacteremia is unknown in 30% of patients.
- **F.** Escherichia coli is the most frequently encountered gram-negative organism, followed by Klebsiella pneumoniae, Enterobacter aerogenes or cloacae, Serratia marcescens, Pseudomonas aeruginosa, Proteus mirabilis, Providencia, and Bacteroides species. Up to 16% of sepsis cases are polymicrobic.
- **G.** Gram-positive organisms, including methicillin-sensitive and methicillin-resistant Staphylococcus aureus and Staphylococcus epidermidis, are associated with catheter or line-related infections.

II. Diagnosis

- **A.** A patient who is hypotensive and in shock should be evaluated to identify the site of infection, and monitor for end-organ dysfunction. History should be obtained and a physical examination performed.
- **B.** **The early phases of septic shock** may produce evidence of volume depletion, such as dry mucous membranes, and cool, clammy skin. After resuscitation with fluids, however, the clinical picture resembles hyperdynamic shock, including tachycardia, bounding pulses with a widened pulse pressure, a hyperdynamic precordium on palpation, and warm extremities.
- **C.** **Signs of infection** include fever, localized erythema or tenderness, consolidation on chest examination, abdominal tenderness, and meningismus. Signs of end-organ hypoperfusion include tachypnea, oliguria, cyanosis, mottling of the skin, digital ischemia, abdominal tenderness, and altered mental status.

D. **Laboratory studies** should include arterial blood gases, lactic acid level, electrolytes, renal function, liver function tests, and chest radiograph. Cultures of blood, urine, and sputum should be obtained before antibiotics are administered. Cultures of pleural, peritoneal, and cerebrospinal fluid may be appropriate. If thrombocytopenia or bleeding is present, tests for disseminated intravascular coagulation should include fibrinogen, d-dimer assay, platelet count, peripheral smear for schistocytes, prothrombin time, and partial thromboplastin time.

Manifestations of Sepsis

Clinical features	Laboratory findings
Temperature instability	Respiratory alkaloses
Tachypnea	Hypoxemia
Hyperventilation	Increased serum lactate levels
Altered mental status	Leukocytosis and increased neutrophil concentration
Oliguria	Eosinopenia
Tachycardia	Thrombocytopenia
Peripheral vasodilation	Anemia
	Proteinuria
	Mildly elevated serum bilirubin levels

III. Treatment of septic shock

A. Early management of septic shock is aimed at restoring mean arterial pressure to 65 to 75 mm Hg to improve organ perfusion. Continuous SVO_2 monitoring is recommended to insure optimal organ perfusion at the cellular level. Clinical clues to adequate tissue perfusion include skin temperature, mental status, and urine output. Urine output should be maintained at >20 to 30 mL/hr. Lactic acid levels should decrease within 24 hours if therapy is effective.

B. **Intravenous access and monitoring**

1. Intravenous access is most rapidly obtained through peripheral sites with two 16- to 18-gauge catheters. More stable access can be achieved later with central intravenous access. Placement of a large-bore introducer catheter in the right internal jugular or left subclavian vein allows the most rapid rate of infusion.

2. Arterial lines should be placed to allow for more reliable monitoring of blood pressure. Pulmonary artery catheters measure cardiac output, systemic vascular resistance, pulmonary artery wedge pressure, and mixed venous oxygen saturation. These data are useful in providing rapid assessment of response to various therapies.

C. **Fluids**

1. Aggressive volume resuscitation is essential in treatment of septic shock. Most patients require 4 to 8 L of crystalloid. Fluid should be administered as a bolus. The mean arterial pressure should be increased to 65 to 75 mm Hg and organ perfusion should be improved within 1 hour of the onset of hypotension.

2. Repeated boluses of crystalloid (isotonic sodium chloride solution or lactated Ringer's injection), 500 to 1,000 mL, should be given intravenously over 5 to 10 minutes, until mean arterial pressure and tissue perfusion are adequate (about 4 to 8 L total over 24 hours for the typical patient). Boluses of 250 mL are appropriate for patients who are elderly or who have heart disease or suspected pulmonary edema.

Red blood cells should be reserved for patients with a hemoglobin value of less than 10 g/dL and either evidence of decreased oxygen delivery or significant risk from anemia (eg, coronary artery disease).

D. Vasoactive agents

1. Patients who do not respond to fluid therapy should receive vasoactive agents. The primary goal is to increase mean arterial pressure to 65 to 75 mm Hg.

2. **Dopamine (Intropin)** traditionally has been used as the initial therapy in hypotension, primarily because it is thought to increase systemic blood pressure. However, dopamine is a relatively weak vasoconstrictor in septic shock.

Hemodynamic effects of vasoactive agents				
Agent	Dose	Effect		
		CO	MAP	SVR
Dopamine (Intropin)	5-20 mcg/kg/min	2+	1+	3+
Norepinephrine (Levophed)	0.05-0.5 mcg/kg/min	-/0/+	2+	4+
Dobutamine (Dobutrex)	10 mcg/kg/min	2+	-/0/+	-/0
Epinephrine	0.05-2 mcg/kg/min	3+	2+	4+
Phenylephrine (Neo-Synephrine)	2-10 mcg/kg/min	0	2+	4+

3. **Norepinephrine (Levophed)** is superior to dopamine in the treatment of hypotension associated with septic shock. Norepinephrine is the agent of choice for treatment of hypotension related to septic shock.

4. **Dobutamine (Dobutrex)** should be reserved for patients with a persistently low cardiac index or underlying left ventricular dysfunction.

E. Antibiotics should be administered within 2 hours of the recognition of sepsis. Use of vancomycin should be restricted to settings in which the causative agent is most likely resistant *Enterococcus,* methicillin-resistant *Staphylococcus aureus,* or high-level penicillin-resistant *Streptococcus pneumoniae.*

Recommended Antibiotics in Septic Shock

Suspected source	Recommended antibiotics
Pneumonia	Third or 4th-generation cephalosporin (cefepime, ceftazidime, cefotaxime, ceftizoxime) *plus* macrolide (antipseudomonal beta lactam *plus* aminoglycoside if hospital-acquired) ± anaerobic coverage with metronidazole or clindamycin.
Urinary tract	Ampicillin *plus* gentamicin (Garamycin) or third-generation cephalosporin (ceftazidime, cefotaxime, ceftizoxime) or a quinolone (ciprofloxacin, levofloxacin).
Skin or soft tissue	Nafcillin (add metronidazole [Flagyl] or clindamycin if anaerobic infection suspected)
Meningitis	Third-generation cephalosporin (ceftazidime, cefotaxime, ceftizoxime)
Intra-abdominal	Third-generation cephalosporin (ceftazidime, cefotaxime, ceftizoxime) *plus* metronidazole or clindamycin
Primary bacteremia	Ticarcillin/clavulanate (Timentin) *or* piperacillin/tazobactam(Zosyn)

Dosages of Antibiotics Used in Sepsis

Agent	Dosage
Cefepime (Maxipime)	2 gm IV q12h; if neutropenic, use 2 gm q8h
Ceftizoxime (Cefizox)	2 gm IV q8h
Ceftazidime (Fortaz)	2 g IV q8h
Cefotaxime (Claforan)	2 gm IV q4-6h
Cefuroxime (Kefurox, Zinacef)	1.5 g IV q8h
Cefoxitin (Mefoxin)	2 gm q6h
Cefotetan (Cefotan)	2 gm IV q12h
Piperacillin/tazobactam (Zosyn)	3.375-4.5 gm IV q6h
Ticarcillin/clavulanate (Timentin)	3.1 gm IV q4-6h (200-300 mg/kg/d)
Ampicillin	1-3.0 gm IV q6h
Ampicillin/sulbactam (Unasyn)	3.0 gm IV q6h
Nafcillin (Nafcil)	2 gm IV q4-6h

Agent	Dosage
Piperacillin, ticarcillin, mezlocillin	3 gm IV q4-6h
Meropenem (Merrem)	1 gm IV q8h
Imipenem/cilastatin (Primaxin)	1.0 gm IV q6h
Gentamicin or tobramycin	2 mg/kg IV loading dose, then 1.7 mg/kg IV q8h
Amikacin (Amikin)	7.5 mg/kg IV loading dose, then 5 mg/kg IV q8h
Vancomycin	1 gm IV q12h
Metronidazole (Flagyl)	500 mg IV q6-8h
Clindamycin (Cleocin)	600-900 mg IV q8h
Linezolid (Zyvox)	600 mg IV/PO q12h
Quinupristin/dalfopristin (Synercid)	7.5 mg/kg IV q8h

1. **Initial treatment of life-threatening sepsis** usually consists of a third or 4th-generation cephalosporin (cefepime, ceftazidime, cefotaxime, ceftizoxime) or piperacillin/tazobactam (Zosyn). An aminoglycoside (gentamicin, tobramycin, or amikacin) should also be included. Antipseudomonal coverage is important for hospital- or institutional-acquired infections. Appropriate choices include an antipseudomonal penicillin, cephalosporin, or an aminoglycoside.

2. **Methicillin-resistant staphylococci.** If line sepsis or an infected implanted device is a possibility, vancomycin should be added to the regimen to cover for methicillin-resistant Staph aureus and methicillin-resistant Staph epidermidis.

3. **Vancomycin-resistant enterococcus (VRE):** An increasing number of enterococcal strains are resistant to ampicillin and gentamicin. The incidence of vancomycin-resistant enterococcus (VRE) is rapidly increasing.

   a. **Linezolid (Zyvox)** is an oral or parenteral agent active against vancomycin-resistant enterococci, including E. faecium and E. faecalis. Linezolid is also active against methicillin-resistant staphylococcus aureus.

   b. **Quinupristin/dalfopristin (Synercid)** is a parenteral agent active against strains of vancomycin-resistant enterococcus faecium, but not enterococcus faecalis. Most strains of VRE are enterococcus faecium.

F. **Other therapies**

1. **Hydrocortisone** (100 mg every 8 hours) in patients with refractory shock significantly improves hemodynamics and survival rates. Corticosteroids may be beneficial in patients with refractory shock caused by an Addison's crisis.

2. **Activated protein C (drotrecogin alfa [Xigris])** has antithrombotic, profibrinolytic, and anti-inflammatory properties. Activated protein C reduces the risk of death by 20%. Activated protein C is approved for treatment of patients with severe sepsis who are at high risk of death. Drotrecogin alfa is administered as 24 mcg/kg/hr for 96 hours. There is a small risk of bleeding. Contraindications are thrombocytopenia, coagulopathy, recent surgery or recent hemorrhage.

Peritonitis

I. Acute Peritonitis

A. Acute peritonitis is inflammation of the peritoneum or peritoneal fluid from bacteria or intestinal contents in the peritoneal cavity. Secondary peritonitis results from perforation of a viscus caused by acute appendicitis or diverticulitis, perforation of an ulcer, or trauma. Primary peritonitis refers to peritonitis arising without a recognizable preceding cause. Tertiary peritonitis consists of persistent intra-abdominal sepsis without a discrete focus of infection, usually occurring after surgical treatment of peritonitis.

B. **Clinical features**

1. Acute peritonitis presents with abdominal pain, abdominal tenderness, and the absence of bowel sounds. Severe, sudden-onset abdominal pain suggests a ruptured viscus. Signs of peritoneal irritation include abdominal tenderness, rebound tenderness, and abdominal rigidity.

2. In severe cases, fever, hypotension, tachycardia, and acidosis may occur. Spontaneous bacterial peritonitis arising from ascites will often present with only subtle signs.

C. **Diagnosis**

1. **Plain abdominal radiographs and a chest x-ray** may detect free air in the abdominal cavity caused by a perforated viscus. CT and/or ultrasonography can identify the presence of free fluid or an abscess.

2. **Paracentesis**

   a. **Tube 1** - Cell count and differential (1-2 mL, EDTA purple top tube)

   b. **Tube 2** - Gram stain of sediment; C&S, AFB, fungal C&S (3-4 mL); inject 10-20 mL into anaerobic and aerobic culture bottle at the bedside.

   c. **Tube 3** - Glucose, protein, albumin, LDH, triglyceride, specific gravity, amylase, (2-3 mL, red top tube). Serum/fluid albumin gradient should be determined.

   d. **Syringe** - pH (3 mL).

D. **Treatment of acute peritonitis**

1. Resuscitation with intravenous fluids and correction of metabolic and electrolyte disturbances are the initial steps. Laparotomy is a corner-stone of therapy for secondary or tertiary acute peritonitis.

2. Broad-spectrum systemic antibiotics are critical to cover bowel flora, including anaerobic species.

3. **Mild to moderate infection (community-acquired)**

   a. Cefotetan (Cefotan) 1-2 gm IV q12h **OR**

   b. Ampicillin/sulbactam (Unasyn) 3.0 gm IV q6h **OR**

   c. Ticarcillin/clavulanate (Timentin) 3.1 gm IV q6h

4. **Severe infection (hospital-acquired)**

   a. Cefepime (Maxipime) 2 gm IV q12h and metronidazole (Flagyl) 500 mg IV q6h **OR**

        b. Piperacillin/tazobactam (Zosyn) 3.375 gm IV q6h **OR**
        c. Imipenem/cilastatin (Primaxin) 1 g IV q6h **OR**
        d. Ciprofloxacin (Cipro) 400 mg IV q12h and clindamycin 600 mg IV q8h **OR**
        e. Gentamicin or tobramycin 100-120 mg (1.5 mg/kg); then 80 mg IV q8h (3-5 mg/kg/d) and metronidazole (Flagyl) 500 mg IV q6h.

II. Spontaneous bacterial peritonitis

A. SBP, which has no obvious precipitating cause, occurs almost exclusively in cirrhotic patients

B. Diagnosis

   1. Spontaneous bacterial peritonitis is diagnosed by paracentesis in which the ascitic fluid is found to have 250 or more polymorphonuclear (PMN) cells per cubic millimeter.

C. Therapy

   1. Antibiotics are the cornerstone of managing SBP, and laparotomy has no place in therapy for SBP, unless perforation is present. Three to 5 days of intravenous treatment with broad-spectrum antibiotics is usually adequate, at which time efficacy can be determined by estimating the ascitic fluid PMN cell count.

   2. Option 1:
      a. Cefotaxime (Claforan) 2 gm IV q4-6h

   3. Option 2:
      a. Ticarcillin/clavulanate (Timentin) 3.1 gm IV q6h **OR**
      b. Piperacillin/tazobactam (Zosyn) 3.375 gm IV q6h or 4.5 gm IV q8h.

   4. Option 3 if extended-spectrum beta-lactamase (ESBL):
      a. Imipenem/cilastatin (Primaxin) 1.0 gm IV q6h. **OR**
      b. Ciprofloxacin (Cipro) 400 mg IV q12h **OR**
      c. Levofloxacin (Levaquin) 500 mg IV q24h.

Gastrointestinal Disorders

Michael Krutzik, MD
H.L. Daneschvar, MD
S.E. Wilson, MD
Roham T. Zamanian, MD

Upper Gastrointestinal Bleeding

When bleeding is believed to be caused by a source proximal to the ligament of Treitz or the source of bleeding is indeterminant, flexible upper gastrointestinal endoscopy is indicated after initial resuscitation and stabilization.

I. **Clinical evaluation**
   A. Initial evaluation of upper GI bleeding should estimate the severity, duration, location, and cause of bleeding. A history of bleeding occurring after forceful vomiting suggests Mallory-Weiss Syndrome.
   B. Abdominal pain, melena, hematochezia (bright red blood per rectum), history of peptic ulcer, cirrhosis or prior bleeding episodes may be present.
   C. **Precipitating factors.** Use of aspirin, nonsteroidal anti-inflammatory drugs, alcohol, or anticoagulants should be sought.

II. **Physical examination**
   A. **General:** Pallor and shallow, rapid respirations may be present; tachycardia indicates a 10% blood volume loss. Postural hypotension (increase in pulse of 20 and a systolic blood pressure fall of 10-15 mmHg), indicates a 20-30% loss.
   B. **Skin:** Delayed capillary refill and stigmata of liver disease (jaundice, spider angiomas, parotid gland hypertrophy) should be sought.
   C. **Abdomen:** Scars, tenderness, masses, hepatomegaly, and dilated abdominal veins should be evaluated. Stool occult blood should be checked.

III. **Laboratory evaluation:** CBC, SMA 12, liver function tests, amylase, INR/PTT, type and cross for pRBC, ECG.

IV. **Differential diagnosis of upper bleeding:** Peptic ulcer, gastritis, esophageal varices, Mallory-Weiss tear, esophagitis, swallowed blood from epistaxis, malignancy (esophageal, gastric), angiodysplasias, aorto-enteric fistula, hematobilia.

V. **Management of upper gastrointestinal bleeding**
   A. If the bleeding appears to have stopped or has significantly slowed, medical therapy with H2 blockers and saline lavage is usually all that is required.
   B. Two 14- to16-gauge IV lines should be placed. Normal saline solution should be infused until blood is ready, then transfuse 2-6 units of pRBCs as fast as possible.
   C. A large bore nasogastric tube should be placed, followed by lavage with 2 L of room temperature tap water. The tube should then be connected to low intermittent suction, and the lavage should be repeated hourly. The NG tube may be removed when bleeding is no longer active.
   D. Oxygen is administered by nasal cannula. Urine output should be monitored.

   E. Serial hematocrits should be checked and maintained greater than 30%. Coagulopathy should be assessed and corrected with fresh frozen plasma, vitamin K, cryoprecipitate, and platelets.
   F. Definitive diagnosis requires upper endoscopy, at which time electrocoagulation, banding, and/or local injection of vasoconstrictors at bleeding sites may be completed. Surgical consultation should be requested in unstable patients or patients who require more than 6 units of pRBCs.

Clinical Indicators of Gastrointestinal Bleeding and Probable Source		
Clinical Indicator	Probability of Upper Gastrointestinal source	Probability of Lower Gastrointestinal Source
Hematemesis	Almost certain	Rare
Melena	Probable	Possible
Hematochezia	Possible	Probable
Blood-streaked stool	Rare	Almost certain
Occult blood in stool	Possible	Possible

VI. Peptic Ulcer Disease
   A. Peptic ulcer disease is the commonest cause of upper gastrointestinal bleeding, responsible for 27-40% of all upper gastrointestinal bleeding episodes. Duodenal ulcer is more frequent than gastric ulcer. Three fourths of all peptic ulcer hemorrhages subside spontaneously.
   B. Upper gastrointestinal endoscopy is the most effective diagnostic technique for peptic ulcer disease. Endoscopic therapy is the method of choice for controlling active ulcer hemorrhage.
   C. **Proton-pump inhibitor administration** is effective in decreasing rebleeding rates with bleeding ulcers. Therapy consists of intravenous pantoprazole.
      1. **Pantoprazole (Protonix)** dosage is 80 mg IV, followed by continuous infusion with 8 mg/hr, then 40 mg PO bid when active bleeding has subsided.
      2. Twice daily dosing of oral proton pump inhibitors may be a reasonable alternative when intravenous formulations are not available. Oral omeprazole (Prilosec) for duodenal ulcer: 20 mg qd for 4-8 weeks. Gastric ulcers: 20 mg bid. Lansoprazole (Prevacid), 15 mg qd. Esomeprazole (Nexium) 20-40 mg qd.
   D. **Indications for surgical operation** include (1) severe hemorrhage unresponsive to initial resuscitative measures; (2) failure of endoscopic or other nonsurgical therapies; and (3) perforation, obstruction, or suspicion of malignancy.
   E. **Duodenal ulcer hemorrhage.** Suture ligation of the ulcer-associated bleeding artery combined with a vagotomy is indicated for duodenal ulcer hemorrhage that does not respond to medical therapy. Truncal vagotomy

and pyloroplasty is widely used because it is rapidly and easily accomplished.

F. **Gastric ulcer hemorrhage** is most often managed by truncal vagotomy and pyloroplasty with wedge excision of ulcer.

G. **Transcatheter angiographic embolization** of the bleeding artery responsible for ulcer hemorrhage is recommended in patients who fail endoscopic attempts at control and who are poor surgical candidates.

VII. Hemorrhagic Gastritis

A. The diffuse mucosal inflammation of gastritis rarely manifest as severe or life-threatening hemorrhage. Hemorrhagic gastritis accounts for 4% of upper gastrointestinal hemorrhage. The bleeding is usually mild and self-limited. When coagulopathy accompanies cirrhosis and portal hypertension, however, gastric mucosal bleeding can be brisk and refractory.

B. Endoscopic therapy can be effective for multiple punctate bleeding sites, but when diffuse mucosal hemorrhage is present, selective intra-arterial infusion of vasopressin may control bleeding. For the rare case in which surgical intervention is required, total gastrectomy is the most effective procedure.

VIII. Mallory-Weiss syndrome

A. This disorder is defined as a mucosal tear at the gastroesophageal junction following forceful retching and vomiting.

B. Treatment is supportive, and the majority of patients stop bleeding spontaneously. Endoscopic coagulation or operative suturing may rarely be necessary.

Esophageal Varices

Esophageal varices eventually develop in most patients with cirrhosis, but variceal bleeding occurs in only one third of them. The initiating event in the development of portal hypertension is increased resistance to portal outflow.

Causes of Portal Hypertension

Presinusoidal
> **Extrahepatic causes**
> Portal vein thrombosis
> Extrinsic compression of the portal vein
> Cavernous transformation of the portal vein
> **Intrahepatic causes**
> Sarcoidosis
> Primary biliary cirrhosis
> Hepatoportal sclerosis
> Schistosomiasis

Sinusoidal: Cirrhosis, alcoholic hepatitis

Postsinusoidal
> Budd-Chiari syndrome (hepatic vein thrombosis)
> Veno-occlusive disease
> Severe congestive heart failure
> Restrictive heart disease

I. Pathophysiology

A. Varices develop annually in 5% to 15% of patients with cirrhosis, and varices enlarge by 4% to 10% each year. Each episode of variceal hemorrhage carries a 20% to 30% risk of death.

B. After an acute variceal hemorrhage, bleeding resolves spontaneously in 50% of patients. Bleeding is least likely to stop in patients with large varices and a Child-Pugh class C cirrhotic liver.

II. Management of variceal hemorrhage

A. **Primary prophylaxis**

1. All patients with cirrhosis should undergo endoscopy to screen for varices every 2 to 3 years.

2. Propranolol (Inderal) and nadolol (Corgard) reduce portal pressure through beta, blockade. Beta-blockade reduces the risk of bleeding by 45% and bleeding-related death by 50%. The beta-blocker dose is adjusted to decrease the resting heart rate by 25% from its baseline, but not to less than 55 to 60 beats/min.

3. Propranolol (Inderal) is given at 10 to 480 mg daily, in divided doses, or nadolol (Corgard) 40 to 320 mg daily in a single dose.

B. **Treatment of acute hemorrhage**

1. Variceal bleeding should be considered in any patient who presents with significant upper gastrointestinal bleeding. Signs of cirrhosis may include spider angiomas, palmar erythema, leukonychia, clubbing, parotid enlargement, and Dupuytren's contracture. Jaundice, lower extremity edema and ascites are indicative of decompensated liver disease.

2. The severity of the bleeding episode can be assessed on the basis of orthostatic changes (eg, resting tachycardia, postural hypotension), which indicates one-third or more of blood volume loss.

3. Blood should be replaced as soon as possible. While blood for transfusion is being made available, intravascular volume should be replenished with normal saline solution. Once euvolemia is established, the intravenous infusion should be changed to solutions with a lower sodium content (5% dextrose with 1/2 or 1/4 normal saline). Blood should be transfused to maintain a hematocrit of at least 30%. Serial hematocrit estimations should be obtained during continued bleeding.

4. Fresh frozen plasma is administered to patients who have been given massive transfusions. Each 3 units of PRBC should be accompanied by $CaCL_2$ 1 gm IV over 30 min. Clotting factors should be assessed. Platelet transfusions are reserved for counts below 50,000/mL in an actively bleeding patient.

5. If the patient's sensorium is altered because of hepatic encephalopathy, the risk of aspiration mandates endotracheal intubation. Placement of a large-caliber nasogastric tube (22 F or 24 F) permits tap water lavage for removal of blood and clots in preparation for endoscopy.

6. **Octreotide acetate (Sandostatin)** is a synthetic, analogue of somatostatin, which causes splanchnic vasoconstriction. Octreotide is the drug of choice in the pharmacologic management of acute variceal bleeding. Octreotide infusion should be started with a loading dose of 50 micrograms, followed by an infusion of 50 micrograms/hr. Treatment is continued until hemorrhage subsides. Definitive endoscopic therapy is performed shortly after hemostasis is achieved.

7. **Endoscopic therapy**
   a. A sclerosant (eg, morrhuate [Scleromate]) is injected into each varix. Complications include bleeding ulcers, dysphagia due to strictures, and pleural effusions.
   b. Endoscopic variceal ligation with elastic bands is an alternative to sclerotherapy because of fewer complications and similar efficacy.
   c. If bleeding persists (or recurs within 48 hours of the initial episode) despite pharmacologic therapy and two endoscopic therapeutic attempts at least 24 hours apart, patients should be considered for salvage therapy with TIPS or surgical treatment (transection of esophageal varices and devascularization of the stomach, portacaval shunt, or liver transplantation).
8. **Transjugular intrahepatic portosystemic shunt (TIPS)** consists of the angiographic creation of a shunt between hepatic and portal veins which is kept open by a fenestrated metal stent. It decompresses the portal system, controlling active variceal bleeding over 90% of the time. Complications include secondary bleeding, worsening encephalopathy in 20%, and stent thrombosis or stenosis.

C. Secondary prophylaxis
1. A patient who has survived an episode of variceal hemorrhage has an overall risk of rebleeding that approaches 70% at 1 year.
2. **Endoscopic sclerotherapy** decreases the risk of rebleeding (50% versus 70%) and death (30% to 60% versus 50% to 75%). Endoscopic variceal ligation is superior to sclerotherapy. Banding is carried out every 2 to 3 weeks until obliteration.

Lower Gastrointestinal Bleeding

The spontaneous remission rates for lower gastrointestinal bleeding is 80 percent. No source of bleeding can be identified in 12 percent of patients, and bleeding is recurrent in 25 percent. Bleeding has usually ceased by the time the patient presents to the emergency room.

I. Clinical evaluation
   A. The severity of blood loss and hemodynamic status should be assessed immediately. Initial management consists of resuscitation with crystalloid solutions (lactated Ringers) and blood products if necessary.
   B. The duration and quantity of bleeding should be assessed; however, the duration of bleeding is often underestimated.
   C. Risk factors that may have contributed to the bleeding include nonsteroidal anti-inflammatory drugs, anticoagulants, colonic diverticulitis, renal failure, coagulopathy, colonic polyps, and hemorrhoids. Patients may have a prior history of hemorrhoids, diverticulosis, inflammatory bowel disease, peptic ulcer, gastritis, cirrhosis, or esophageal varices.
   D. **Hematochezia.** Bright red or maroon output per rectum suggests a lower GI source; however, 12 to 20% of patients with an upper GI bleed may have hematochezia as a result of rapid blood loss.
   E. **Melena.** Sticky, black, foul-smelling stools suggest a source proximal to the ligament of Treitz, but Melena can also result from bleeding in the small intestine or proximal colon.

F. **Clinical findings**
1. **Abdominal pain** may result from ischemic bowel, inflammatory bowel disease, or a ruptured aneurysm.
2. **Painless massive bleeding** suggests vascular bleeding from diverticula, angiodysplasia, or hemorrhoids.
3. **Bloody diarrhea** suggests inflammatory bowel disease or an infectious origin.
4. **Bleeding with rectal pain** is seen with anal fissures, hemorrhoids, and rectal ulcers.
5. **Chronic constipation** suggests hemorrhoidal bleeding. New onset of constipation or thin stools suggests a left sided colonic malignancy.
6. **Blood on the toilet paper** or dripping into the toilet water suggests a perianal source of bleeding, such as hemorrhoids or an anal fissure.
7. **Blood coating** the outside of stools suggests a lesion in the anal canal.
8. **Blood streaking** or mixed in with the stool may results from polyps or a malignancy in the descending colon.
9. **Maroon colored stools** often indicate small bowel and proximal colon bleeding.

II. **Physical examination**
A. **Postural hypotension** indicates a 20% blood volume loss, whereas, overt signs of shock (pallor, hypotension, tachycardia) indicates a 30 to 40 percent blood loss.
B. **The skin** may be cool and pale with delayed refill if bleeding has been significant.
C. **Stigmata of liver disease**, including jaundice, caput medusae, gynecomastia and palmar erythema, should be sought because patients with these findings frequently have GI bleeding.

III. **Differential diagnosis of lower GI bleeding**
A. **Angiodysplasia** and diverticular disease of the right colon accounts for the vast majority of episodes of acute lower GI bleeding. Most acute lower GI bleeding originates from the colon however 15 to 20 percent of episodes arise from the small intestine and the upper GI tract.
B. **Elderly patients.** Diverticulosis and angiodysplasia are the most common causes of lower GI bleeding.
C. **Younger patients.** Hemorrhoids, anal fissures and inflammatory bowel disease are most common causes of lower GI bleeding.

Clinical Indicators of Gastrointestinal Bleeding and Probable Source		
Clinical Indicator	**Probability of Upper Gastrointestinal source**	**Probability of Lower Gastrointestinal Source**
Hematemesis	Almost certain	Rare
Melena	Probable	Possible
Hematochezia	Possible	Probable
Blood-streaked stool	Rare	Almost certain
Occult blood in stool	Possible	Possible

IV. **Diagnosis and management of lower gastrointestinal bleeding**
   A. **Rapid clinical evaluation and resuscitation** should precede diagnostic studies. Intravenous fluids (1 to 2 liters) should be infused over 10- 20 minutes to restore intravascular volume, and blood should be transfused if there is rapid ongoing blood loss or if hypotension or tachycardia are present. Coagulopathy is corrected with fresh frozen plasma, platelets, and cryoprecipitate.
   B. When small amounts of bright red blood are passed per rectum, then lower GI tract can be assumed to be the source. In patients with large volume maroon stools, nasogastric tube aspiration should be performed to exclude massive upper gastrointestinal hemorrhage.
   C. If the nasogastric aspirate contains no blood then anoscopy and sigmoidoscopy should be performed to determine weather a colonic mucosal abnormality (ischemic or infectious colitis) or hemorrhoids might be the cause of bleeding.
   D. **Colonoscopy** in a patient with massive lower GI bleeding is often nondiagnostic, but it can detect ulcerative colitis, antibiotic-associated colitis, or ischemic colon.
   E. **Polyethylene glycol-electrolyte solution** (CoLyte or GoLytely) should be administered by means of a nasogastric tube (Four liters of solution is given over a 2-3 hour period), allowing for diagnostic and therapeutic colonoscopy.

V. **Definitive management of lower gastrointestinal bleeding**
   A. **Colonoscopy**
      1. Colonoscopy is the procedure of choice for diagnosing colonic causes of GI bleeding. It should be performed after adequate preparation of the bowel. If the bowel cannot be adequately prepared because of persistent, acute bleeding, a bleeding scan or angiography is preferable.
      2. If colonoscopy fails to reveal the source of the bleeding, the patient should be observed because, in 80% of cases, bleeding ceases spontaneously.
   B. **Radionuclide scan or bleeding scan.** Technetium- labeled (tagged) red blood cell bleeding scans can detect bleeding sites when bleeding is intermittent. Localization may not he a precise enough to allow segmental colon resection.
   C. **Angiography**. Selective mesenteric angiography detects arterial bleeding that occurs at rates of 0.5 mL/per minute or faster. Diverticular bleeding causes pooling of contrast medium within a diverticulum. Bleeding angiodysplastic lesions appear as abnormal vasculature. When active bleeding is seen with diverticular disease or angiodysplasia, selective arterial infusion of vasopressin may be effective.
   D. **Surgery**
      1. If bleeding continues and no source can be found, surgical intervention is usually warranted. Surgical resection may be indicated for patients with recurrent diverticular bleeding, or for patients who have had persistent bleeding from colonic angiodysplasia and have required blood transfusions.
      2. Surgical management of lower gastrointestinal bleeding is ideally undertaken with a secure knowledge of the location and cause of the bleeding lesion. A segmental bowel resection to include the lesion and followed by a primary anastomosis is usually safe and appropriate in all but the most unstable patients.

VI. Diverticulosis

A. Diverticulosis of the colon is present in more than 50% of the population by age 60 years. Bleeding from diverticula is relatively rare, affecting only 4% to 17% of patients at risk.

B. In most cases, bleeding ceases spontaneously, but in 10% to 20% of cases, the bleeding continues. The risk of rebleeding after an episode of bleeding is 25%. Right-sided colonic diverticula occur less frequently than left-sided or sigmoid diverticula but are responsible for a disproportionate incidence of diverticular bleeding.

C. Operative management of diverticular bleeding is indicated when bleeding continues and is not amenable to angiographic or endoscopic therapy. It also should be considered in patients with recurrent bleeding in the same colonic segment. The operation usually consists of a segmental bowel resection (usually a right colectomy or sigmoid colectomy) followed by a primary anastomosis.

VII. Arteriovenous malformations

A. AVMs or angiodysplasias are vascular lesions that occur primarily in the distal ileum, cecum, and ascending colon of elderly patients. The arteriographic criteria for identification of an AVM include a cluster of small arteries, visualization of a vascular tuft, and early and prolonged filling of the draining vein.

B. The typical pattern of bleeding of an AVM is recurrent and episodic, with most individual bleeding episodes being self-limited. Anemia is frequent, and continued massive bleeding is distinctly uncommon. After nondiagnostic colonoscopy, enteroscopy should be considered.

C. Endoscopic therapy for AVMs may include heater probe, laser, bipolar electrocoagulation, or argon beam coagulation. Operative management is usually reserved for patients with continued bleeding, anemia, repetitive transfusion requirements, and failure of endoscopic management. Surgical management consists of segmental bowel resection with primary anastomosis.

VIII. Inflammatory bowel disease

A. Ulcerative colitis and, less frequently, Crohn's colitis or enteritis may present with major or massive lower gastrointestinal bleeding. Infectious colitis can also manifest with bleeding, although it is rarely massive.

B. When the bleeding is minor to moderate, therapy directed at the inflammatory condition is appropriate. When the bleeding is major and causes hemodynamic instability, surgical intervention is usually required. When operative intervention is indicated, the patient is explored through a midline laparotomy, and a total abdominal colectomy with end ileostomy and oversewing of the distal rectal stump is the preferred procedure.

IX. Tumors of the colon and rectum

A. Colon and rectal tumors account for 5% to 10% of all hospitalizations for lower gastrointestinal bleeding. Visible bleeding from a benign colonic or rectal polyp is distinctly unusual. Major or massive hemorrhage rarely is caused by a colorectal neoplasm; however, chronic bleeding is common. When the neoplasm is in the right colon, bleeding is often occult and manifests as weakness or anemia.

B. More distal neoplasms are often initially confused with hemorrhoidal bleeding. For this reason, the treatment of hemorrhoids should always be preceded by flexible sigmoidoscopy in patients older than age 40 or 50 years. In younger patients, treatment of hemorrhoids without further investigation may be appropriate if there are no risk factors for neoplasm, there is a consistent clinical history, and there is anoscopic evidence of recent bleeding from enlarged internal hemorrhoids.

X. Anorectal disease

A. When bleeding occurs only with bowel movements and is visible on the toilet tissue or the surface of the stool, it is designated *outlet bleeding*. Outlet bleeding is most often associated with internal hemorrhoids or anal fissures.

B. Anal fissures are most commonly seen in young patients and are associated with severe pain during and after defecation. Other benign anorectal bleeding sources are proctitis secondary to inflammatory bowel disease, infection, or radiation injury. Additionally, stercoral ulcers can develop in patients with chronic constipation.

C. Surgery for anorectal problems is typically undertaken only after failure of conservative medical therapy with high-fiber diets, stool softeners, and/or hemorrhoidectomy.

XI. Ischemic colitis

A. Ischemic colitis is seen in elderly patients with known vascular disease. The abdomen pain may be postprandial and associated with bloody diarrhea or rectal bleeding. Severe blood loss is unusual but can occur.

B. Abdominal films may reveal "thumb-printing" caused by submucosal edema. Colonoscopy reveals a well-demarcated area of hyperemia, edema and mucosal ulcerations. The splenic flexure and descending colon are the most common sites. Most episodes resolve spontaneously, however, vascular bypass or resection may be required.

Acute Pancreatitis

The incidence of acute pancreatitis ranges from 54 to 238 episodes per 1 million per year. Patients with mild pancreatitis respond well to conservative therapy, but those with severe pancreatitis may have a progressively downhill course to respiratory failure, sepsis, and death (less than 10%).

I. Etiology

A. **Alcohol-induced pancreatitis.** Consumption of large quantities of alcohol may cause acute pancreatitis.

B. **Cholelithiasis.** Common bile duct or pancreatic duct obstruction by a stone may cause acute pancreatitis. (90% of all cases of pancreatitis occur secondary to alcohol consumption or cholelithiasis).

C. **Idiopathic pancreatitis.** The cause of pancreatitis cannot be determined in 10 percent of patients.

D. **Hypertriglyceridemia.** Elevation of serum triglycerides (>I,000mg/dL) has been linked with acute pancreatitis.

E. **Pancreatic duct disruption.** In younger patients, a malformation of the pancreatic ducts (eg, pancreatic divisum) with subsequent obstruction is often the cause of pancreatitis. In older patients without an apparent underlying etiology, cancerous lesions of the ampulla of Vater, pancreas or duodenum must be ruled out as possible causes of obstructive pancreatitis.

F. **Iatrogenic pancreatitis.** Radiocontrast studies of the hepatobiliary system (eg, cholangiogram, ERCP) can cause acute pancreatitis in 2-3% of patients undergoing studies.

G. **Trauma.** Blunt or penetrating trauma of any kind to the peri-pancreatic or peri-hepatic regions may induce acute pancreatitis. Extensive surgical manipulation can also induce pancreatitis during laparotomy.

Causes of Acute Pancreatitis	
Alcoholism Cholelithiasis Drugs Hypertriglyceridemia Idiopathic causes	Infections Microlithiasis Pancreas divisum Trauma

Medications Associated with Acute Pancreatitis	
Definitive Association: Azathioprine (Imuran) Sulfonamides Thiazide diuretics Furosemide (Lasix) Estrogens Tetracyclines Valproic acid (Depakote) Pentamidine Didanosine (Videx)	**Probable Association:** Acetaminophen Nitrofurantoin Methyldopa Erythromycin Salicylates Metronidazole NSAIDS ACE-inhibitors

II. **Pathophysiology.** Acute pancreatitis results when an initiating event causes the extrusion of zymogen granules, from pancreatic acinar cells, into the interstitium of the pancreas. Zymogen particles cause the activation of trypsinogen into trypsin. Trypsin causes auto-digestion of pancreatic tissues.

III. **Clinical presentation**
   A. **Signs and symptoms.** Pancreatitis usually presents with mid-epigastric pain that radiates to the back, associated with nausea and vomiting. The pain is sudden in onset, progressively increases in intensity, and becomes constant. The severity of pain often causes the patient to move continuously in search of a more comfortable position.
   B. **Physical examination**
      1. Patients with acute pancreatitis often appear very ill. Findings that suggest severe pancreatitis include hypotension and tachypnea with decreased basilar breath sounds. Flank ecchymoses (Grey Tuner's Sign) or periumbilical ecchymoses (Cullen's sign) may be indicative of hemorrhagic pancreatitis.
      2. Abdominal distension and tenderness in the epigastrium are common. Fever and tachycardia are often present. Guarding, rebound tenderness, and hypoactive or absent bowel sounds indicate peritoneal irritation. Deep palpation of abdominal organs should be avoided in the setting of suspected pancreatitis.

IV. **Laboratory testing**
   A. **Leukocytosis.** An elevated WBC with a left shift and elevated hematocrit (indicating hemoconcentration) and hyperglycemia are common. Pre-renal azotemia may result from dehydration. Hypoalbuminemia, hypertriglyceridemia, hypocalcemia, hyperbilirubinemia, and mild elevations of transaminases and alkaline phosphatase are common.
   B. **Elevated amylase.** An elevated amylase level often confirms the clinical diagnosis of pancreatitis.

C. **Elevated lipase.** Lipase measurements are more specific for pancreatitis than amylase levels, but less sensitive. Hyperlipasemia may also occur in patients with renal failure, perforated ulcer disease, bowel infarction and bowel obstruction.

D. **Abdominal Radiographs** may reveal non-specific findings of pancreatitis, such as "sentinel loops" (dilated loops of small bowel in the vicinity of the pancreas), ileus and, pancreatic calcifications.

E. **Ultrasonography** demonstrates the entire pancreas in only 20 percent of patients with acute pancreatitis. Its greatest utility is in evaluation of patients with possible gallstone disease.

F. **Helical high resolution computed tomography** is the imaging modality of choice in acute pancreatitis. CT findings will be normal in 14-29% of patients with mild pancreatitis. Pancreatic necrosis, pseudocysts and abscesses are readily detected by CT.

Selected Conditions Other Than Pancreatitis Associated with Amylase Elevation	
Carcinoma of the pancreas	Acute alcoholism
Common bile duct obstruction	Diabetic ketoacidosis
Post-ERCP	Lung cancer
Mesenteric infarction	Ovarian neoplasm
Pancreatic trauma	Renal failure
Perforated viscus	Ruptured ectopic pregnancy
Renal failure	Salivary gland infection
	Macroamylasemia

V. **Prognosis.** Ranson's criteria is used to determine prognosis in acute pancreatitis. Patients with two or fewer risk factors have a mortality rate of less than 1 percent, those with three or four risk-factors a mortality rate of 16 percent, five or six risk factors, a mortality rate of 40 percent, and seven or eight risk factors, a mortality rate approaching 100 percent.

Ranson's Criteria for Acute Pancreatitis	
At admission	**During initial 48 hours**
1. Age >55 years	1. Hematocrit drop >10%
2. WBC >16,000/mm^3	2. BUN rise >5 mg/dL
3. Blood glucose >200 mg/dL	3. Arterial pO$_2$ <60 mm Hg
4. Serum LDH >350 IU/L	4. Base deficit >4 mEq/L
5. AST >250 U/L	5. Serum calcium <8.0 mg/dL
	6. Estimated fluid sequestration >6 L

VI. **Treatment of pancreatitis**

A. **Expectant management.** Most cases of acute pancreatitis will improve within three to seven days. Management consists of prevention of complications of severe pancreatitis.

B. **NPO and bowel rest.** Patients should take nothing by mouth. Total parenteral nutrition should be instituted for those patients fasting for more than five days. A nasogastric tube is warranted if vomiting or ileus.

    C. **IV fluid resuscitation.** Vigorous intravenous hydration is necessary. A decrease in urine output to less than 30 mL per hour is an indication of inadequate fluid replacement.

    D. **Pain control.** Morphine is discouraged because it may cause Oddi's sphincter spasm, which may exacerbate the pancreatitis. Meperidine (Demerol), 25-100 mg IV/IM q4-6h, is favored. Ketorolac (Toradol), 60 mg IM/IV, then 15-30 mg IM/IV q6h, is also used.

    E. **Antibiotics.** Routine use of antibiotics is not recommended in most cases of acute pancreatitis. In cases of infectious pancreatitis, treatment with cefoxitin (1-2 g IV q6h), cefotetan (1-2 g IV q12h), imipenem (1.0 gm IV q6h), or ampicillin/sulbactam (1.5-3.0 g IV q6h) may be appropriate.

    F. **Alcohol withdrawal prophylaxis.** Alcoholics may require alcohol withdrawal prophylaxis with lorazepam (Ativan) 1-2mg IM/IV q4-6h as needed x 3 days, thiamine 100mg IM/IV qd x 3 days, folic acid 1 mg IM/IV qd x 3 days, multivitamin qd.

    G. **Octreotide.** Somatostatin is also a potent inhibitor of pancreatic exocrine secretion. Octreotide is a somatostatin analogue, which has been effective in reducing mortality from bile-induced pancreatitis. Clinical trials, however, have failed to document a significant reduction in mortality

    H. **Blood sugar monitoring and insulin administration.** Serum glucose levels should be monitored.

VII. **Complications**

    A. Chronic pancreatitis

    B. Severe hemorrhagic pancreatitis

    C. Pancreatic pseudocysts

    D. Infectious pancreatitis with development of sepsis (occurs in up to 5% of all patients with pancreatitis)

    E. Portal vein thrombosis

Hepatic Encephalopathy

Hepatic encephalopathy develops when ammonia and toxins, which are usually metabolized (detoxified) by the liver, enter into the systemic circulation. Hepatic encephalopathy can be diagnosed in 50-70% of patients with chronic hepatic failure.

I. **Clinical manifestations**

    A. Hepatic encephalopathy manifests as mild changes in personality to altered motor functions and/or level of consciousness.

    B. Most episodes are precipitated by identifiable factors, including gastrointestinal bleeding, excessive protein intake, constipation, excessive diuresis, hypokalemia, hyponatremia or hypernatremia, azotemia, infection, poor compliance with lactulose therapy, sedatives (benzodiazepines, barbiturates, antiemetics), hepatic insult (alcohol, drugs, viral hepatitis), surgery, or hepatocellular carcinoma.

C. **Hepatic encephalopathy** is a diagnosis of exclusion. Therefore, if a patient with acute or chronic liver failure suddenly develops altered mental status, concomitant problems must be excluded, such as intracranial lesions (hemorrhage, infarct, tumor, abscess), infections (meningitis, encephalitis, sepsis), metabolic encephalopathies (hyperglycemia or hypoglycemia, uremia, electrolyte imbalance), alcohol intoxication or withdrawal, Wernicke's encephalopathy, drug toxicity (sedatives, psychoactive medications), or postictal encephalopathy.

D. **Physical exam** may reveal hepatosplenomegaly, ascites, jaundice, spider angiomas, gynecomastia, testicular atrophy, and asterixis.

E. **Computed tomography** may be useful to exclude intracranial abscess or hemorrhage. Laboratory evaluation may include serum ammonia, CBC, electrolyte panel, liver profile, INR/PTT, UA, and blood cultures.

II. Treatment of hepatic encephalopathy

A. **Flumazenil (Romazicon)** may transiently improve the mental state in patients with hepatic encephalopathy. Dosage is 0.2 mg (2 mL) IV over 30 seconds q1min until a total dose of 3 mg; if a partial response occurs, continue 0.5 mg doses until a total of 5 mg. Excessive doses of flumazenil may precipitate seizures.

B. **Lactulose** is a non-absorbable disaccharide, which decreases the absorption of ammonia into the blood stream. Lactulose can be given orally, through a nasogastric tube, or rectally (less effective). The dosage is 30-45 mL PO q1h x 3 doses, then 15-45 mL PO bid-qid titrate to produce 2-4 soft stools/d. A laxative such as magnesium sulfate and an enema are given before lactulose therapy is started. Lactulose enema (300 mL of lactulose in 700 mL of tap water), 250 mL PR q6h.

C. **Neomycin**, a poorly absorbed antibiotic, alters intestinal flora and reduces the release of ammonia into the blood (initially 1-2 g orally four times a day). Because chronic neomycin use can cause nephrotoxicity and ototoxicity, neomycin should be used for short periods of time, and the dose should be decreased to 1-2 g/day after achievement of the desired clinical effect. Alternatively, metronidazole can be given at 250 mg orally three times a day alone or with neomycin.

D. **Dietary protein** is initially withheld, and intravenous glucose is administered to prevent excessive endogenous protein breakdown. As the patient improves, dietary protein can be reinstated at a level of 20 gm per day and then increased gradually to a minimum of 60 gm per day. If adequate oral intake of protein cannot be achieved, therapy with oral or enteral formulas of casein hydrolysates (Ensure) or amino acids (FreAmine) is indicated.

References: See page 168.

Toxicologic Disorders

Hans Poggemeyer, MD

Poisoning and Drug Overdose

I. **Management of poisoning and drug overdose**
   A. Stabilize vital signs; maintain airway, breathing and circulation.
   B. Consider intubation if patient has depressed mental status and is at risk for aspiration or respiratory failure.
   C. Establish IV access and administer oxygen.
   D. Draw blood for baseline labs (see below).
   E. If altered mental status is present, administer D50W 50 mL IV push, followed by naloxone (Narcan) 2 mg IV, followed by thiamine 100 mg IV.

II. **Gastrointestinal decontamination**
   A. **Gastric lavage**
      1. Studies have challenged the safety and efficacy of gastric lavage. Lavage retrieves less than 30% of the toxic agent when performed 1 hour after ingestion. Gastric lavage may propel toxins into the duodenum, and accidental placement of the tube into the trachea or mainstem bronchus may occur.
      2. Gastric lavage may be considered if the patient has ingested a potentially life-threatening amount of poison and the procedure can be undertaken within 60 minutes of ingestion.
      3. **Contraindications:** Acid, alkali, or hydrocarbons.
      4. Place the patient in Trendelenburg's position and left lateral decubitus. Insert a large bore (32-40) french Ewald orogastric tube. A smaller NG tube may be used but may be less effective in retrieving large particles.
      5. After tube placement has been confirmed by auscultation, aspirate stomach contents and lavage with 200 cc aliquots of saline or water until clear (up to 2 L). The first 100 cc of fluid should be sent for toxicology analysis.
   B. **Activated charcoal**
      1. Activated charcoal is not effective for alcohols, aliphatic hydrocarbons, caustics, cyanide, elemental metals (boric acid, iron, lithium, lead), or pesticides.
      2. The oral or nasogastric dose is 50 gm mixed with sorbitol. The dose should be repeated at 25-50 gm q4-6h for 24-48 hours if massive ingestion, sustained release products, tricyclic antidepressants, phenothiazines, sertraline (Zoloft), paroxetine (Paxil), carbamazepine, digoxin, phenobarbital, phenytoin, valproate, salicylate, doxepin, or theophylline were ingested.
      3. Give oral cathartic (70% sorbitol) with charcoal.
   C. **Whole bowel irrigation**
      1. Whole bowel irrigation can prevent further absorption in cases of massive ingestion, delayed presentation, or in overdoses of enteric coated or sustained release pills. This treatment may be useful in eliminating objects, such as batteries, or ingested packets of drugs.
      2. Administer GoLytely, or CoLyte orally at 1.6-2.0 liter per hour until fecal effluent is clear.

D. **Hemodialysis:** Indications include ingestion of phenobarbital, theophylline, chloral hydrate, salicylate, ethanol, lithium, ethylene glycol, isopropyl alcohol, procainamide, and methanol, or severe metabolic acidosis.

E. **Hemoperfusion:** May be more effective than hemodialysis **except** for bromides, heavy metals, lithium, and ethylene glycol. Hemoperfusion is effective for disopyramide, phenytoin, barbiturates, theophylline.

Toxicologic Syndromes

I. **Characteristics of common toxicologic syndromes**

A. **Cholinergic poisoning:** Salivation, bradycardia, defecation, lacrimation, emesis, urination, miosis.

B. **Anticholinergic poisoning:** Dry skin, flushing, fever, urinary retention, mydriasis, thirst, delirium, conduction delays, tachycardia, ileus.

C. **Sympathomimetic poisoning:** Agitation, hypertension, seizure, tachycardia, mydriasis, vasoconstriction.

D. **Narcotic poisoning:** Lethargy, hypotension, hypoventilation, miosis, coma, ileus.

E. **Withdrawal syndrome:** Diarrhea, lacrimation, mydriasis, cramps, tachycardia, hallucination.

F. **Salicylate poisoning:** Fever, respiratory alkalosis, or mixed acid-base disturbance, hyperpnea, hypokalemia, tinnitus.

G. **Causes of toxic seizures:** Amoxapine, anticholinergics, camphor, carbon monoxide, cocaine, ergotamine, isoniazid, lead, lindane, lithium, LSD, parathion, phencyclidine, phenothiazines, propoxyphene propranolol, strychnine, theophylline, tricyclic antidepressants, normeperidine (metabolite of meperidine), thiocyanate.

H. **Causes of toxic cardiac arrhythmias:** Arsenic, beta-blockers, chloral hydrate, chloroquine, clonidine, calcium channel blockers, cocaine, cyanide, carbon monoxide, digitalis, ethanol, phenol, phenothiazine, tricyclics.

I. **Extrapyramidal syndromes:** Dysphagia, dysphonia, trismus, rigidity, torticollis, laryngospasm.

Acetaminophen Overdose

I. **Clinical features**

A. Acute lethal dose = 13-25 g. Acetaminophen is partly metabolized to N-acetyl-p-benzoquinonimine which is conjugated by glutathione. Hepatic glutathione stores can be depleted in acetaminophen overdose, leading to centrilobular hepatic necrosis.

B. Liver failure occurs 3 days after ingestion if untreated. Liver failure presents with right upper quadrant pain, elevated liver function tests, coagulopathy, hypoglycemia, renal failure and encephalopathy.

II. **Treatment**

A. **Gastrointestinal decontamination** should consist of gastric lavage followed by activated charcoal. Residual charcoal should be removed with saline lavage prior to giving N-acetyl-cysteine (NAC).

B. Check acetaminophen level 4 hours after ingestion. A nomogram should be used to determine if treatment is necessary (see next page). Start treatment if level is above the nontoxic range or if the level is potentially toxic but the time of ingestion is unknown.

C. Therapy must start no later than 8-12 hours after ingestion. Treatment after 16-24 hours of non-sustained release formulation is significantly less effective, but should still be accomplished.

D. Oral N-acetyl-cysteine (Mucomyst): 140 mg/kg PO followed by 70 mg/kg PO q4h x 17 doses (total 1330 mg/kg over 72 h). Repeat loading dose if emesis occurs. Complete all doses even after acetaminophen level falls below critical value.

E. Hemodialysis and hemoperfusion are somewhat effective, but should not take the place of NAC treatment.

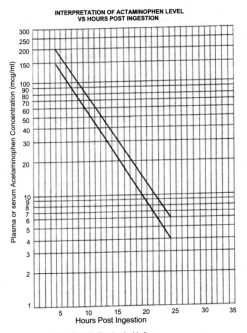

INTERPRETATION OF ACTAMINOPHEN LEVEL VS HOURS POST INGESTION

No risk of toxicity if under double lines.
Probable risk if above top line.
Possible risk if between double lines.
Outcome is best if treatment is initiated within 12 hours of ingestion.
Graph applies to non-sustained release formulations only .

Cocaine Overdose

I. Clinical evaluation

A. Cocaine can be used intravenously, smoked, ingested, or inhaled nasally. Street cocaine often is cut with other substances including amphetamines, LSD, PCP, heroin, strychnine, lidocaine, talc, and quinine.

B. One-third of fatalities occur within 1 hour, with another third occurring 6-24 hours later.

C. Persons may transport cocaine by swallowing wrapped packets, and some users may hastily swallow packets of cocaine to avoid arrest.

II. Clinical features

A. **CNS:** Sympathetic stimulation, agitation, seizures, tremor, headache, subarachnoid hemorrhage, ischemic cerebral stoke, psychosis, hallucinations, fever, mydriasis, formication (sensation of insects crawling on skin).

B. **Cardiovascular:** Atrial and ventricular arrhythmias, myocardial infarction, hypertension, hypotension, myocarditis, aortic rupture, cardiomyopathy.

C. **Pulmonary:** Noncardiogenic pulmonary edema, pneumomediastinum, alveolar hemorrhage, hypersensitivity pneumonitis, bronchiolitis obliterans.

D. **Other:** Rhabdomyolysis, mesenteric ischemia, hepatitis.

III. Treatment

A. Treatment consists of supportive care because no antidote exists. GI decontamination, including repeated activated charcoal, whole bowel irrigation and endoscopic evaluation is provided if oral ingestion is suspected.

B. Hyperadrenergic symptoms should be treated with benzodiazepines, such as lorazepam.

C. **Seizures:** Treat with lorazepam, phenytoin, or phenobarbital.

D. **Arrhythmias**
   1. Treat hyperadrenergic state and supraventricular tachycardia with lorazepam and propranolol.
   2. Ventricular arrhythmias are treated with lidocaine or propranolol.

E. **Hypertension**
   1. Use lorazepam first for tachycardia and hypertension.
   2. If no response, use labetalol because it has alpha and beta blocking effects.
   3. If hypertension remains severe, administer sodium nitroprusside or esmolol drip.

F. **Myocardial ischemia and infarction:** Treat with thrombolysis, heparin, aspirin, beta-blockers, nitroglycerin. Control hypertension and exclude CNS bleeding before using thrombolytic therapy.

Cyclic Antidepressant Overdose

I. Clinical features

A. Antidepressants have prolonged body clearance rates, and cannot be removal by forced diuresis, hemodialysis, and hemoperfusion. Delayed absorption is common because of decreased GI motility from anticholinergic effects. Cyclic antidepressants undergo extensive enterohepatic recirculation.

B. **CNS:** Lethargy, coma, hallucinations, seizures, myoclonic jerks.

C. **Anticholinergic crises:** Blurred vision, dilated pupils, urinary retention, dry mouth, ileus, hyperthermia.
D. **Cardiac:** Hypotension, ventricular tachyarrhythmias, sinus tachycardia.
E. **ECG:** Sinus tachycardia, right bundle branch block, right axis deviation, increased PR and QT interval, QRS >100 msec, or right axis deviation. Prolongation of the QRS width is a more reliable predictor of CNS and cardiac toxicity than the serum level.

II. Treatment
A. Gastrointestinal decontamination and systemic drug removal
1. Magnesium citrate 300 mL via nasogastric tube x 1 dose.
2. Activated charcoal premixed with sorbitol 50 gm via nasogastric tube q4-6h around-the-clock until the serum level decreases to therapeutic range. Maintain the head-of-bed at a 30-45 degree angle to prevent aspiration.
3. **Cardiac toxicity**
   a. Alkalinization is a cardioprotective measure and it has no influence on drug elimination. The goal of treatment is to achieve an arterial pH of 7.50-7.55. If mechanical ventilation is necessary, hyperventilate to maintain desired pH.
   b. Administer sodium bicarbonate 50-100 mEq (1-2 amps or 1-2 mEq/kg) IV over 5-10 min. Followed by infusion of sodium bicarbonate, 2 amps in 1 liter of D5W at 100-150 cc/h. Adjust IV rate to maintain desired pH.
4. **Seizures**
   a. Administer lorazepam or diazepam IV followed by phenytoin.
   b. Physostigmine, 1-2 mg slow IV over 3-4 min, is necessary if seizures continue.

Digoxin Overdose

I. Clinical features
A. The therapeutic window of digoxin is 0.8-2.0 ng/mL. Drugs that increase digoxin levels include verapamil, quinidine, amiodarone, flecainide, erythromycin, and tetracycline. Hypokalemia, hypomagnesemia and hypercalcemia enhance digoxin toxicity.
B. **CNS:** Confusion, lethargy; yellow-green visual halo.
C. **Cardiac:** Common dysrhythmias include ventricular tachycardia or fibrillation; variable atrioventricular block, atrioventricular dissociation; sinus bradycardia, junctional tachycardia, premature ventricular contractions.
D. **GI:** Nausea, vomiting.
E. **Metabolic:** Hypokalemia enhances the toxic effects of digoxin on the myocardial tissue and may be present in patients on diuretics.

II. Treatment
A. **Gastrointestinal decontamination:** Gastric lavage, followed by repeated doses of activated charcoal, is effective; hemodialysis is ineffective.
B. Treat bradycardia with atropine, isoproterenol, and cardiac pacing.
C. Treat ventricular arrhythmias with lidocaine or phenytoin. Avoid procainamide and quinidine because they are proarrhythmic and slow AV conduction.
D. Electrical DC cardioversion may be dangerous in severe toxicity. Hypomagnesemia and hypokalemia should be corrected.

E. **Digibind (Digoxin-specific Fab antibody fragment)**
   1. Indication: Life-threatening arrhythmias refractory to conventional therapy.
   2. Dosage of Digoxin immune Fab:

   (number of 40 mg vials)= $\dfrac{\text{Digoxin level (ng/mL) x body weight (kg)}}{100}$

   3. Dissolve the digoxin immune Fab in 100-150 mL of NS and infuse IV over 15-30 minutes. A 0.22 micron in-line filter should be used during infusion.
   4. Hypokalemia, heart failure, and anaphylaxis may occur. The complex is renally excreted; after administration, serum digoxin levels may be artificially high because both free and bound digoxin is measured.

Ethylene Glycol Ingestion

I. **Clinical features**
   A. **Ethylene glycol** is found in antifreeze, detergents, and polishes.
   B. **Toxicity:** Half-life 3-5 hours; the half-life increases to 17 hours if coingested with alcohol. The minimal lethal dose is 1.0-1.5 cc/kg, and the lethal blood level is 200 mg/dL.
   C. Anion gap metabolic acidosis and severe osmolar gap is often present. CNS depression and cranial nerve dysfunction (facial and vestibulocochlear palsies) are common.
   D. GI symptoms such as flank pain. Oxalate crystals may be seen in the urine sediment. Other findings may include hypocalcemia (due to calcium oxalate formation); tetany, seizures, and prolonged QT.

II. **Treatment**
   A. Fomepizole (Antizol) loading dose 15 mg/kg IV; then 10 mg/kg IV q12h x 4, then 15 mg/kg IV q12h until ethylene glycol level is <20 mg/dL.
   B. Pyridoxine 100 mg IV qid x 2 days and thiamine 100 mg IV qid x 2 days.
   C. If definitive therapy is not immediately available, 3-4 ounces of whiskey (or equivalent) may be given orally.
   D. **Hemodialysis indications:** Severe refractory metabolic acidosis, crystalluria, serum ethylene glycol level >50 mg/dL; keep glycol level <10 mg/dL.

Gamma-hydroxybutyrate Ingestion

I. **Clinical features**
   A. Gamma-hydroxybutyrate (GHB) was used as an anesthetic agent but was banned because of the occurrence of seizures. Gamma-hydroxybutyrate is now an abused substance at dance clubs because of the euphoric effects of the drug. It is also abused by body builders because of a mistaken belief that it has anabolic properties. Gamma-hydroxybutyrate is a clear, odorless, oily, salty liquid. It is rapidly absorbed within 20-40 minutes of ingestion and metabolized in the liver. The half-life of GHB is 20-30 min.
   B. Gamma-hydroxybutyrate is not routinely included on toxicological screens, but it can be detected in the blood and urine by gas chromatography

within 12 hours of ingestion. Gamma hydroxybutyrate may cause respiratory depression, coma, seizures, and severe agitation. Cardiac effects include hypotension, cardiac arrest, and severe vomiting.

II. Treatment
A. Gastric lavage is not indicated due to rapid absorption of GHB.
B. Immediate care consists of support of ventilation and circulation. Agitation should be treated with benzodiazepines, haloperidol, or propofol. Seizures should be treated with lorazepam, phenytoin, or valproic acid.

Iron Overdose

I. Clinical features
A. Toxicity is caused by free radical organ damage to the GI mucosa, liver, kidney, heart, and lungs. The cause of death is usually shock and liver failure.

Toxic dosages and serum levels	
Nontoxic	<10-20 mg/kg of elemental iron (0-100 mcg/dL)
Toxic	>20 mg/kg of elemental iron (350-1000 mcg/dL)
Lethal	>180-300 mg/kg of elemental iron (>1000 mcg/dL)

B. **Two hours after ingestion:** Severe hemorrhagic gastritis; vomiting, diarrhea, lethargy, tachycardia, and hypotension.
C. **Twelve hours after ingestion:** Improvement and stabilization.
D. **12-48 hours after ingestion:** GI bleeding, coma, seizures, pulmonary edema, circulatory collapse, hepatic and renal failure, coagulopathy, hypoglycemia, and severe metabolic acidosis.

II. Treatment
A. Administer deferoxamine if iron levels reach toxic values. Deferoxamine 100 mg binds 9 mg of free elemental iron. The deferoxamine dosage is 10-15 mg/kg/hr IV infusion.
B. Treat until 24 hours after vin rose colored urine clears. Serum iron levels during chelation are not accurate. Deferoxamine can cause hypotension, allergic reactions such as pruritus, urticarial wheals, rash, anaphylaxis, tachycardia, fever, and leg cramps.
C. **Gastrointestinal decontamination**
   1. Charcoal is not effective in absorbing elemental iron. Abdominal x-rays should be evaluated for remaining iron tablets. Consider whole bowel lavage if iron pills are past the stomach and cannot be removed by gastric lavage (see page 128).
   2. **Hemodialysis** is indicated for severe toxicity.

Isopropyl Alcohol Ingestion

I. **Clinical features**
   A. **Isopropyl alcohol** is found in rubbing alcohol, solvents, and antifreeze.
   B. **Toxicity:** Lethal dose: 3-4 g/kg
      1. Lethal blood level: 400 mg/dL
      2. Half-life = 3 hours
   C. **Metabolism:** Isopropyl alcohol is metabolized to acetone. Toxicity is characterized by an anion gap metabolic acidosis with high serum ketone level; mild osmolar gap; mildly elevated glucose.
   D. CNS depression, headache, nystagmus; cardiovascular depression, abdominal pain and vomiting, and pulmonary edema may occur.

II. **Treatment**
   A. Treatment consists of supportive care. No antidote is available; ethanol is not indicated.
   B. **Hemodialysis:** Indications: refractory hypotension, coma, potentially lethal blood levels.

Lithium Overdose

I. **Clinical features**
   A. Lithium has a narrow therapeutic window of 0.8-1.2 mEq/L.
   B. Drugs that will increase lithium level include NSAIDs, phenothiazines, thiazide and loop diuretics (by causing hyponatremia).
   C. **Toxicity**
      1.5-3.0 mEq/L = moderate toxicity
      3.0-4.0 mEq/L = severe toxicity
   D. Toxicity in chronic lithium users occurs at much lower serum levels than with acute ingestions.
   E. Common manifestations include seizures, encephalopathy, hyperreflexia, tremor, nausea, vomiting, diarrhea, hypotension. Nephrogenic diabetes insipidus and hypothyroidism may also occur. Conduction block and dysrhythmias are rare, but reversible T-wave depression may occur.

II. **Treatment**
   A. Correct hyponatremia with aggressive normal saline hydration. Follow lithium levels until <1.0 mEq/L.
   B. **Forced solute diuresis:** Hydrate with normal saline infusion to maintain urine output at 2-4 cc/kg/hr; use furosemide (Lasix) 40-80 mg IV doses as needed.
   C. **Gastrointestinal decontamination**
      1. Administer gastric lavage. Activated charcoal is ineffective. Whole bowel irrigation may be useful.
      2. **Indications for hemodialysis:** Level >4 mEq/L; CNS or cardiovascular impairment with level of 2.5-4.0 mEq/L.

Methanol Ingestion

I. **Clinical features**
   A. **Methanol** is found in antifreeze, Sterno, cleaners, and paints.

    B. Toxicity
        1. 10 cc causes blindness
        2. Minimal lethal dose = 1-5 g/kg
        3. Lethal blood level = 80 mg/dL
        4. Symptomatic in 40 minutes to 72 hours.

    C. Signs and Symptoms
        1. Severe osmolar and anion gap metabolic acidosis.
        2. Visual changes occur because of optic nerve toxicity, leading to blindness.
        3. Nausea, vomiting, abdominal pain, pancreatitis, and altered mental status.

II. Treatment
    A. Ethanol 10% is infuse in D5W as 7.5 cc/kg load then 1.4 cc/kg/h drip to keep blood alcohol level between 100-150 mg/dL. Continue therapy until the methanol level is below 20-25 mg/dL.
    B. Give folate 50 mg IV q4h to enhance formic acid metabolism.
    C. Correct acidosis and electrolyte imbalances.
    D. Hemodialysis: Indications: peak methanol level >50 mg/dL; formic acid level >20 mg/dL; severe metabolic acidosis; acute renal failure; any visual compromise.

Salicylate Overdose

I. Clinical features
    A. Toxicity
        150-300 mg/kg - mild toxicity
        300-500 mg/kg - moderate toxicity
        >500 mg/kg - severe toxicity
    B. Chronic use can cause toxicity at much lower levels (ie, 25 mg/dL) than occurs with acute use.
    C. Acid/Base Abnormalities: Patients present initially with a respiratory alkalosis because of central hyperventilation. Later an anion gap metabolic acidosis occurs.
    D. CNS: Tinnitus, lethargy, irritability, seizures, coma, cerebral edema.
    E. GI: Nausea, vomiting, liver failure, GI bleeding.
    F. Cardiac: Hypotension, sinus tachycardia, AV block, wide complex tachycardia.
    G. Pulmonary: Non-cardiogenic pulmonary edema, adult respiratory distress syndrome.
    H. Metabolic: Renal failure; coagulopathy because of decreased factor VII; hyperthermia because of uncoupled oxidative phosphorylation. Hypoglycemia may occur in children, but it is rare in adults.

II. Treatment
    A. Provide supportive care and GI decontamination. Aspirin may form concretions or drug bezoars, and ingestion of enteric coated preparations may lead to delayed toxicity.
    B. Multiple dose activated charcoal, whole bowel irrigation, and serial salicylate levels are indicated. Hypotension should be treated vigorously with fluids. Abnormalities should be corrected, especially hypokalemia. Urine output should be maintained at 200 cc/h or more. Metabolic acidosis should be treated with bicarbonate 50-100 mEq (1-2 amps) IVP.

C. Renal clearance is increased by alkalinization of urine with a bicarbonate infusion (2-3 amps in 1 liter of D5W IV at 150-200 mL/h), keeping the urine pH at 7.5-8.5.

D. **Hemodialysis** is indicated for seizures, cardiac or renal failure, intractable acidosis, acute salicylate level >120 mg/dL or chronic level >50 mg/dL (therapeutic level 15-25 mg/dL).

Theophylline Toxicity

I. Clinical features

A. Drug interactions can increase serum theophylline level, including quinolone and macrolide antibiotics, propranolol, cimetidine, and oral contraceptives. Liver disease or heart failure will decrease clearance.

B. **Serum toxicity levels**
20-40 mg/dL - mild
40-70 mg/dL - moderate
>70 mg/dL - life threatening

C. Toxicity in chronic users occurs at lower serum levels than with short-term users. Seizures and arrhythmias can occur at therapeutic or minimally supra-therapeutic levels.

D. **CNS:** Hyperventilation, agitation, and tonic-clonic seizures.

E. **Cardiac:** Sinus tachycardia, multi-focal atrial tachycardia, supraventricular tachycardia, ventricular tachycardia and fibrillation, premature ventricular contractions, hypotension or hypertension.

F. **Gastrointestinal:** Vomiting, diarrhea, hematemesis.

G. **Musculoskeletal:** Tremor, myoclonic jerks

H. **Metabolic:** Hypokalemia, hypomagnesemia, hypophosphatemia, hyper-glycemia, and hypercalcemia.

II. Treatment

A. **Gastrointestinal decontamination and systemic drug removal**

1. Activated charcoal premixed with sorbitol, 50 gm PO or via nasogastric tube q4h around-the-clock until theophylline level is less than 20 mcg/mL. Maintain head-of-bed at 30 degrees to prevent charcoal aspiration.

2. Hemodialysis is as effective as repeated oral doses of activated charcoal and should be used when charcoal hemoperfusion is not fea-sible.

3. **Indications for charcoal hemoperfusion:** Coma, seizures, hemodynamic instability, theophylline level >60 mcg/mL; rebound in serum levels may occur after discontinuation of hemoperfusion.

4. **Seizures** are generally refractory to anticonvulsants. High doses of lorazepam, diazepam or phenobarbital should be used; phenytoin is less effective.

5. **Treatment of hypotension**
   a. Normal saline fluid bolus.
   b. Norepinephrine 8-12 mcg/min IV infusion or
   c. Phenylephrine 20-200 mcg/min IV infusion.

6. **Treatment of ventricular arrhythmias**
   a. Amiodarone 150-300 mg IV over 10 min, then 1 mg/min x 6 hours, followed by 0.5 mg/min IV infusion. Lidocaine should be avoided because it has epileptogenic properties.

b. Esmolol (Brevibloc) 500 mcg/kg/min loading dose, then 50-300 mcg/kg/min continuous IV drip.

Warfarin (Coumadin) Overdose

I. Clinical management

A. Elimination measures: Gastric lavage and activated charcoal if recent oral ingestion of warfarin (Coumadin).

B. Reversal of coumadin anticoagulation: Coagulopathy should be corrected rapidly or slowly depending on the following factors: 1) Intensity of hypocoagulability, 2) severity or risk of bleeding, 3) need for reinstitution of anticoagulation.

C. Emergent reversal

1. Fresh frozen plasma: Replace vitamin K dependent factors with FFP 2-4 units; repeat in 4 hours if prothrombin time remains prolonged.

2. Vitamin K, 25 mg in 50 cc NS, to infuse no faster than 1 mg/min; risk of anaphylactoid reactions and shock; slow infusion minimizes risk.

D. Reversal over 24-48 Hours: Vitamin K 10-25 mg subcutaneously. Full reversal of anticoagulation will result in resistance to further Coumadin therapy for several days.

E. Partial correction: Lower dose vitamin K (0.5-1.0 mg) will lower prothrombin time without interfering with reinitiation of Coumadin.

References: See page 168.

Neurologic Disorders

Hans Poggemeyer, MD

Acute Ischemic Stroke

I. **Initial general assessment.** Sudden loss of focal brain function is the core feature of the onset of ischemic stroke. The goals in this initial phase include:
   A. Medically stabilize the patient.
   B. Reverse any conditions that are contributing to the patient's problem.
   C. Assess the pathophysiologic basis of the neurologic symptoms.
   D. Screen for potential contraindications to thrombolysis in acute ischemic stroke patients.
   E. Diagnosing an intracerebral hemorrhage (ICH) or subarachnoid hemorrhage (SAH) as soon as possible can be lifesaving. The presence of onset headache and vomiting favor the diagnosis of ICH or SAH compared with a thromboembolic stroke, while the abrupt onset of impaired cerebral function without focal symptoms favors the diagnosis of SAH.
   F. **History and physical examination** should distinguish between seizures, syncope, migraine, and hypoglycemia, which can mimic acute ischemia. In patients with focal signs and altered level of consciousness, it is important to determine whether the patient takes insulin or oral hypoglycemic agents, has a history of a seizure disorder or drug overdose or abuse, medications on admission, or recent trauma.

Acute stroke differential diagnosis

Migraine
Intracerebral hemorrhage
Head trauma
Brain tumor
Todd's palsy (paresis, aphasia, neglect, etc., after a seizure episode)
Functional deficit (conversion reaction)
Systemic infection
Toxic-metabolic disturbances (hypoglycemia, acute renal failure, hepatic insufficiency, exogenous drug
   intoxication)

   G. **Physical examination** should evaluate the neck and retroorbital regions for vascular bruits, and palpate of pulses in the neck, arms, and legs to assess for their absence, asymmetry, or irregular rate.
   1. The heart should be auscultated for murmurs. Fluctuations in blood pressure occasionally precede fluctuations in clinical signs.
   2. The skin should be examined for signs of endocarditis, cholesterol emboli, purpura, or ecchymoses. The funduscopic examination may reveal cholesterol emboli or papilledema. The head should be examined for signs of trauma. A tongue laceration may occur during a seizure.
   3. The neck should be immobilized until evaluated radiographically for evidence of serious trauma if there is a suspicion of a fall. The chest x-ray is helpful if it shows cardiomegaly, metastases, or a widened

mediastinum suggesting aortic dissection. Examination of the extremities is important to detect deep vein thrombosis.

4. **Breathing.** Patients with increased ICP due to hemorrhage, vertebrobasilar ischemia, or bihemispheric ischemia can present with a decreased respiratory drive or muscular airway obstruction. Intubation may be necessary to restore adequate ventilation. Patients with adequate ventilation should have the oxygen saturation monitored. Patients who are hypoxic should receive supplemental oxygen.

H. Immediate laboratory studies

1. All patients with acute neurologic deterioration or acute stroke should have an electrocardiogram. Chest radiography is indicated if lung or heart disease is suspected. Oxygen saturation or arterial blood gas tests are indicated if hypoxia is suspected.

2. **Blood studies include:**
   a. Complete blood count including platelets, and erythrocyte sedimentation rate.
   b. Electrolytes, urea nitrogen, creatinine.
   c. Serum glucose. Finger stick for faster glucose measurement if diabetic, taking insulin or oral hypoglycemic agents, or if there is clinical suspicion for hypoglycemia.
   d. Liver function tests.
   e. Prothrombin time and partial thromboplastin time.
   f. Toxicology screen and blood alcohol level in selected patients.
   g. Blood for type and cross match in case fresh frozen is needed to reverse a coagulopathy if ICH is present.
   h. Urine human chorionic gonadotropin in women of child-bearing potential.
   i. Consider evaluation for hypercoagulable state in young patients without apparent stroke risk factors.

Laboratory studies

Complete blood count and erythrocyte sedimentation rate
Electrolytes, urea nitrogen, creatinine, glucose
Liver function tests
Prothrombin time and partial thromboplastin time
Toxicology screen
Blood for type and cross match
Urine human chorionic gonadotropin in women of child-bearing potential
Consider evaluation for hypercoagulable state in young patients without apparent stroke risk factors

---

3. Anticoagulant use is a common cause of intracerebral hemorrhage. Thus, the prothrombin and partial thromboplastin time and the platelet count should be checked. The effects of warfarin are corrected with intravenous vitamin K and fresh-frozen plasma (typically 4 units) in patients with intracerebral hemorrhage.

4. A drug overdose can mimic an acute stroke. In addition, cocaine, intravenous drug abuse, and amphetamines can cause an ischemic stroke or intracranial hemorrhage. Hyponatremia and thrombotic thrombocytopenic purpura (TTP) can present with focal neurologic deficits, suggesting the need for measurement of serum electrolytes and a complete blood count with platelet count.

5. **Hyperglycemia,** defined as a blood glucose level >108 mg/dL, is associated with poor functional outcome from acute stroke at presentation. Stress hyperglycemia is common in stroke patients, although newly diagnosed diabetes may be detected. Treatment with fluids and insulin to reduce serum glucose to less than 300 mg/dL is recommended.

6. **Hypoglycemia** can cause focal neurologic deficits mimicking stroke. The blood sugar should be checked and rapidly corrected if low. Glucose should be administered immediately after drawing a blood sample in "stroke" patients known to take insulin or oral hypoglycemic agents.

7. **Fever.** Primary central nervous system infection, such as meningitis, subdural empyema, brain abscess, and infective endocarditis, need to be excluded as the etiology of fever. Common etiologies of fever include aspiration pneumonia and urinary tract infection. Fever may contribute to brain injury in patients with an acute stroke. Maintaining normothermia is recommended after an acute stroke. Prophylactic administration of acetaminophen (1 g four times daily) is more effective in preventing fever than placebo (5 versus 36 percent).

8. **Blood pressure management.** Acute management of blood pressure (BP) may vary according to the type of stroke.
   a. **Ischemic stroke.** Blood pressure should not be treated acutely in the patient with ischemic stroke unless the hypertension is extreme (diastolic BP above 120 mm Hg and/or systolic BP above 220 mm Hg), or the patient has active ischemic coronary disease, heart failure, or aortic dissection. If pharmacologic therapy is given, intravenous labetalol is the drug of choice.
   b. **Intracranial hemorrhage.** With ICH, intravenous labetalol, nitroprusside, or nicardipine, should be given if the systolic pressure is above 170 mm Hg. The goal is to maintain the systolic pressure between 140 and 160 mm Hg. Intravenous labetalol is the first drug of choice in the acute phase since it allows rapid titration.

I. **Neurologic evaluation.** The history should focus upon the time of symptom onset, the course of symptoms over time, possible embolic sources, items in the differential diagnosis, and concomitant diseases. The neurologic examination should attempt to confirm the findings from the history and provide a quantifiable examination for further assessment over time.

J. **Neuroimaging** studies are used to exclude hemorrhage as a cause of the deficit, to assess the degree of brain injury, and to identify the vascular lesion responsible for the ischemic deficit.

1. **Computed tomography.** In the hyperacute phase, a non-contrast CT (NCCT) scan is usually ordered to exclude or confirm hemorrhage. A NCCT scan should be obtained as soon as the patient is medically stable.
   a. **Noncontrast CT.** Early signs of infarction include: Subtle parenchymal hypodensity, which can be detected in 45 to 85 percent of cases. Early focal brain swelling is present in up to 40 percent of patients with early infarction and also has been adversely related to outcome. A hyperdense middle cerebral artery (MCA) can be visualized in 30 to 40 percent of patients with an MCA distribution stroke, indicating the presence of thrombus inside the artery lumen (bright artery sign).

2. **Transcranial Doppler ultrasound (TCD)** visualizes intracranial vessels of the circle of Willis. It is a noninvasive means of assessing the patency of intracranial vessels.
3. **Carotid duplex ultrasound** is as a noninvasive examination to evaluate extracranial atherosclerotic disease. It may help to establish the source of an embolic stroke, but is not used acutely.

Initial management of acute stroke

Determine whether stroke is ischemic or hemorrhagic by computed tomography
Consider administration of t-PA if less than three hours from stroke onset
General management:
- Blood pressure (avoid hypotension)
- Assure adequate oxygenation
- Administer intravenous glucose
- Take dysphagia/aspiration precautions
- Consider prophylaxis for venous thrombosis if the patient is unable to walk
- Suppress fever, if present
- Assess stroke mechanism (eg, atrial fibrillation, hypertension)
- Consider aspirin or clopidogrel (Plavix) therapy if ischemic stroke and no contra-indications (begin 24 hours after t-PA).

Antiplatelet Agents for Prevention of Ischemic Stoke

- Enteric-coated aspirin (Ecotrin) 325 mg PO qd
- Clopidogrel (Plavix) 75 mg PO qd
- Extended-release aspirin 25 mg with dipyridamole 200 mg (Aggrenox) one tab PO qd

Eligibility criteria for the treatment of acute ischemic stroke with recombinant tissue plasminogen activator (rt-PA)

Inclusion criteria
Clinical diagnosis of ischemic stroke, with the onset of symptoms within three hours of the initiation of treatment (if the exact time of stroke onset is not know, it is defined as the last time the patient was known to be normal), and with a measurable neurologic deficit.

Exclusion criteria
Historical
    Stroke or head trauma within the prior 3 months
    Any prior history of intracranial hemorrhage
    Major surgery within 14 days
    Gastrointestinal or genitourinary bleeding within the previous 21 days

Clinical
Rapid improving stroke symptoms
Only minor and isolated neurologic signs
Seizure at the onset of stroke with postictal residual neurologic impairments
Symptoms suggestive of subarachnoid hemorrhage, even if the CT is normal
Clinical presentation consistent with acute MI or post-MI pericarditis
Persistent systolic BP >185 diastolic >110 mm Hg, or requiring aggressive therapy to control BP
Pregnancy or lactation
Active bleeding or acute trauma (fracture)

Laboratory
Platelets <100,000/mm^3
Serum glucose <50 mg/dL or >400 mg/dL
INR >1.5 if on warfarin
Elevated partial thromboplastin time if on heparin

Head CT scan
Evidence of hemorrhage
Evidence major early infarct signs, such as diffuse swelling of the affected hemisphere, parenchymal hypodensity, and /or effacement of >35 percent of the middle cerebral artery territory

K. Thrombolytic therapy. Patients presenting within three hours of symptom onset may be given IV alteplase (Activase) (0.9 mg/kg up to 90 mg; 10 percent as a bolus, then a 60 minute infusion).

Elevated Intracranial Pressure

Cerebrospinal fluid (CSF) pressure in excess of 250 mm CSF is usually a manifestation of serious neurologic disease. Intracranial hypertension is most often associated with rapidly expanding mass lesions, CSF outflow obstruction, or cerebral venous congestion.

I. Clinical evaluation
   A. Increased intracranial pressure may manifest as headache caused by traction on pain-sensitive cerebral blood vessels or dura mater.
   B. Papilledema is the most reliable sign of ICP, although it fails to develop in many patients with increased ICP. Retinal venous pulsations, when present, imply that CSF pressure is normal or not significantly elevated. Patients with increased ICP often complain of worsening headache, in the morning.

Causes of Increased Intracranial Pressure	
Diffuse cerebral edema	**Space-occupying lesions**
Meningitis	Intracerebral hemorrhage
Encephalitis	Epidural hemorrhage
Hepatic encephalopathy	Subdural hemorrhage
Reye's syndrome	Tumor
Acute liver failure	Abscess
Electrolyte shifts	**Hydrocephalus**
Dialysis	Subarachnoid hemorrhage
Hypertensive encephalopathy	Meningitis
Posthypoxic brain injury	Aqueductal stenosis
Lead encephalopathy	Idiopathic
Uncompensated hypercarbia	**Miscellaneous**
Head trauma	Pseudotumor cerebri
Diffuse axonal injury	Craniosynostosis
	Venous sinus thrombosis

II. Intracranial pressure monitoring

A. Clinical signs of elevated ICP, such as the Cushing response (systemic hypertension, bradycardia, and irregular respirations), are usually a late findings and may never even occur; therefore, ICP should be directly measured with an invasive device.

B. Normal intracranial pressures range from approximately 10-20 cm H_2O (or about 5 to 15 mm Hg). Ventricular catheterization involves insertion of a sterile catheter into the lateral ventricle.

Treatment of Elevated Intracranial Pressure			
Treatment	**Dose**	**Advantages**	**Limitations**
Hypocarbia by hyperventilation	pCO_2 25 to 33 mm Hg respiratory rate of 10 to 16/min	Immediate onset, well tolerated	Hypotension, barotrauma, duration usually hours or less
Osmotic	Mannitol 0.5 to 1 g/kg IV push	Rapid onset, titratable, predictable	Hypotension, hypokalemia, duration hours or days
Barbiturates	Pentobarbital 25 mg/kg slow IV infusion over 3-4 hours	Mutes BP and respiratory fluctuations	Hypotension, fixed pupils (small), duration days
Hemicraniectomy	Timing critical	Large sustained ICP reduction	Surgical risk, tissue herniation through wound

III. Treatment of increased intracranial pressure

A. **Positioning** the patient in an upright position with the head of the bed at 30 degrees will lower ICP.

B. **Hyperventilation** is the most rapid and effective means of lowering ICP, but the effects are short lived because the body quickly compensates. The pCO_2 should be maintained between 25-33 mm Hg

C. **Mannitol** can quickly lower ICP, although the effect is not long lasting and may lead to dehydration or electrolyte imbalance. Dosage is 0.5-1 gm/kg (37.5-50 gm) IV q6h; keep osmolarity <315; do not give for more than 48h.

D. **Corticosteroids** are best used to treat increased ICP in the setting of vasogenic edema caused by brain tumors or abscesses; however, these agents have little value in the setting of stroke or head trauma. Dosage is dexamethasone (Decadron) 10 mg IV or IM, followed by 4-6 mg IV, IM or PO q6h.

E. **Barbiturate coma** is used for medically intractable ICP elevation when other medical therapies have failed. There is a reduction in ICP by decreasing cerebral metabolism. The pentobarbital loading dose is 25 mg/kg body weight over 3-4 hours, followed by 2-3 mg/kg/hr IV infusion. Blood levels are periodically checked and adjusted to 30-40 mg/dL. Patients require mechanical ventilation, intracranial pressure monitoring, and continuous electroencephalographic monitoring.

F. **Management of blood pressure.** Beta-blockers or mixed beta and alpha blockers provide the best antihypertensive effects without causing significant cerebral vasodilatation that can lead to elevated ICP.

Management of Status Epilepticus

An estimated 152,000 cases of status epilepticus occur per year in the United States, resulting in 42,000 deaths per year. Status epilepticus is defined as two or more sequential seizures without full recovery of consciousness between seizures, or more than 30 minutes of continuous seizure activity. Practically speaking, any person who exhibits persistent seizure activity or who does not regain consciousness for five minutes or more after a witnessed seizure should be considered to have status epilepticus. Status epilepticus is classified into generalized (tonic-clonic, myoclonic, absence, atonic, akinetic) and partial (simple or complex) status epilepticus.

I. **Epidemiology**

A. Status epilepticus of partial onset accounts for the majority of episodes. 69 percent of episodes in adults and 64 percent of episodes in children are partial onset, followed by secondarily generalized status epilepticus in 43 percent of adults and 36 percent of children. The incidence of status epilepticus is bimodally distributed, occurring most frequently during the first year of life and after the age of 60 years. A variety in adults, the major causes were low levels of antiepileptic drugs (34 percent) and cerebrovascular disease (22 percent), including acute or remote stroke and hemorrhage.

Systemic Complications of Generalized Convulsive Status Epilepticus	
Metabolic Lactic acidosis Hypercapnia Hypoglycemia Hyperkalemia Hyponatremia CSF/serum leukocytosis **Autonomic** Hyperpyrexia Failure of cerebral autoregulation Vomiting Incontinence	**Renal** Acute renal failure from rhabdomyolysis Myoglobinuria **Cardiac/respiratory** Hypoxia Arrhythmia High output failure Pneumonia

II. Management of Status Epilepticus

A. A single generalized seizure with complete recovery does not require treatment. Once the diagnosis of status epilepticus is made, however, treatment should be initiated immediately.

B. Physicians first should assess the patient's airway and oxygenation. If the airway is clear and intubation is not immediately required, blood pressure and pulse should be checked and oxygen administered. In patients with a history of seizures, an attempt should be made to determine whether medications have been taken recently. A screening neurologic examination should be performed to check for signs of a focal intracranial lesion.

C. Intravenous access should be obtained, and blood should be sent to the laboratory for measurement of serum electrolyte, blood urea nitrogen, glucose, and antiepileptic drug levels, as well as a toxic drug screen and complete blood cell count. An isotonic saline infusion should be initiated.

D. Glucose, 50 mL of 50 percent, should be given immediately if hypoglycemia is suspected because hypoglycemia may precipitate status epilepticus and is quickly reversible. If the physician cannot check for hypoglycemia or there is any doubt, glucose should be administered empirically. Thiamine (100 mg) should be given along with the glucose, because glucose infusion increases the risk of Wernicke's encephalopathy in susceptible patients.

E. Blood gas levels should be determined to ensure adequate oxygenation. Initially, acidosis, hyperpyrexia, and hypertension need not be treated, because these are common findings in early status epilepticus and should resolve on their own with general treatment. If seizures persist after initial measures, medication should be administered. Imaging with computed tomography is recommended after stabilization of the airway and circulation. If imaging is negative, lumbar puncture is required to rule out infectious etiologies.

III. Electroencephalography

A. Electroencephalography (EEG) is extremely useful in the diagnosis and management of status epilepticus. EEG can establish the diagnosis in less obvious circumstances.

B. EEG also can help to confirm that an episode of status epilepticus has ended. Patients with status epilepticus who fail to recover rapidly and completely should be monitored with EEG for at least 24 hours after an episode.

IV. Pharmacologic management

A. Benzodiazepines

1. The benzodiazepines are some of the most effective drugs in the treatment of acute seizures and status epilepticus. The benzodiazepines most commonly used to treat status epilepticus are diazepam (Valium), lorazepam (Ativan), and midazolam (Versed).

2. **Lorazepam (Ativan)**

   a. Lorazepam has emerged as the preferred benzodiazepine for acute management of status epilepticus. Lorazepam is less lipid-soluble than diazepam, with a distribution half-life of two to three hours versus 15 minutes for diazepam. Therefore, it has a longer duration of clinical effect. Lorazepam also binds the GABAergic receptor more tightly than diazepam, resulting in a longer duration of action.

   b. Anticonvulsant effects of lorazepam last six to 12 hours, and the typical dose ranges from 4 to 8 mg (0.1 mg/kg). Lorazepam has a broad spectrum of efficacy, terminating seizures in 75 to 80 percent of cases. Adverse effects include respiratory suppression, hypotension, sedation, and local tissue irritation.

3. **Phenytoin**

   a. Phenytoin (Dilantin) is one of the most effective drugs for treating acute seizures and status epilepticus. In addition, it is effective in the management of chronic epilepsy.

   b. The main advantage of phenytoin is the lack of a significant sedating effect. Arrhythmias and hypotension have been reported with the IV formulation. These effects are associated with a more rapid rate of administration and the propylene glycol vehicle used as its diluent. In addition, local irritation, phlebitis, and dizziness may accompany intravenous administration.

Antiepileptic Drugs Used in Status Epilepticus

Drug	Loading dose	Maintenance dosage	Adverse effects
Lorazepam (Ativan)	4-8 mg	None	Respiratory depression, hypotension, sialorrhea
Phenytoin (Dilantin)	15 to 18 mg per kg at 50 mg per minute	5 mg per kg per day	Cardiac depression, hypotension
Fosphenytoin (Cerebyx)	18 to 20 mg per kg phenytoin equivalents at 150 mg per minute	4-6 mg PE/kg/day	Cardiac depression, hypotension, paresthesias
Phenobarbital	20 mg per kg	2 mg per kg/kg IV q12h	Respiratory suppression

Drug	Loading dose	Maintenance dosage	Adverse effects
Pentobarbital	10 mg per kg	1-1.5 mg per kg per hour	Hypotension, respiratory suppression
Midazolam (Versed)	0.2 mg per kg	0.05 to 0.6 mg per kg per hour	Hypotension, respiratory suppression
Propofol (Diprivan)	2 mg per kg	5 to 10 mg per kg per hour initially, then 2-10 mg/kg/hr	Respiratory depression, hypotension, lipemia, acidosis

4. Fosphenytoin

   a. Fosphenytoin (Cerebyx) is a water-soluble pro-drug of phenytoin that completely converts to phenytoin. Thus, the adverse events that are related to propylene glycol are avoided. Like phenytoin, fosphenytoin is useful in treating acute partial and generalized tonic-clonic seizures. Fosphenytoin is converted to phenytoin within eight to 15 minutes. Because 1.5 mg of fosphenytoin is equivalent to 1 mg of phenytoin, the dosage, concentration, and infusion rate of intravenous fosphenytoin are expressed as phenytoin equivalents (PE).

Protocol for Management of Status Epilepticus

At: zero minutes
Initiate general systemic support of the airway (insert nasal airway or intubate if needed)

I. Check blood pressure.

II. Begin nasal oxygen.

III. Monitor ECG and respiration.

IV. Check temperature frequently.

V. Obtain history.

VI. Perform neurologic examination.

Send sample serum for evaluation of electrolytes, blood urea nitrogen, glucose level, complete blood cell count, toxic drug screen, and anticonvulsant levels; check arterial blood gas values.
Start IV line containing isotonic saline at a low infusion rate.
Inject 50 mL of 50 percent glucose IV and 100 mg of thiamine IV.
Call EEG laboratory to start recording as soon as feasible.
Administer lorazepam (Ativan) at 0.1 to 0.15 mg per kg IV (2 mg per minute); if seizures persist, administer fosphenytoin (Cerebyx) at 18 mg per kg IV (150 mg per minute, with an additional 7 mg per kg if seizures continue).

At: 20 to 30 minutes, if seizures persist
Intubate, insert bladder catheter, start EEG recording, check temperature.
Administer phenobarbital in a loading dose of 20 mg per kg IV (100 mg per minute).

At: 40 to 60 minutes, if seizures persist
Begin pentobarbital infusion at 5 mg per kg IV initial dose, then IV push until seizures have stopped, using EEG monitoring; continue pentobarbital infusion at 1 mg per kg per hour; slow infusion rate every four to six hours to determine if seizures have stopped, with EEG guidance; monitor blood pressure and respiration carefully. Support blood pressure with pressors if needed.
or
Begin midazolam (Versed) at 0.2 mg per kg, then at a dosage of 0.05-0.6 mg/kg/min, titrated to EEG monitoring.
or
Begin propofol (Diprivan) at 1 to 2 mg per kg loading dose, followed by 2 to 10 mg per kg per hour. Adjust maintenance dosage on the basis of EEG monitoring.

    b. The initial dose of fosphenytoin is 15 to 20 mg PE per kg, given at 150 mg PE per minute. Fosphenytoin may be administered IV or IM, although IM administration has a 3-hour delayed peak effect.

c. Adverse effects that are unique to fosphenytoin include perineal paresthesias and pruritus. Unlike phenytoin, fosphenytoin does not cause local irritation. Intravenous therapy has been associated with hypotension, so continuous cardiac and blood pressure monitoring are recommended.

5. Phenobarbital

a. Phenobarbital is used after lorazepam or phenytoin has failed to control status epilepticus. The normal loading dose is 15 to 20 mg per kg. Because high-dose phenobarbital is sedating, airway protection is important, and aspiration is a major concern. Intravenous phenobarbital also is associated with hypotension. It is diluted in 60 to 80 percent propylene glycol, which is associated with renal failure, myocardial depression, and seizures.

Endocrinologic and Nephrologic Disorders

Michael Krutzik, MD
Guy Foster, MD

Diabetic Ketoacidosis

Diabetic ketoacidosis is defined by hyperglycemia, metabolic acidosis, and ketosis.

I. **Clinical presentation**
   A. Diabetes is newly diagnosed in 20% of cases of diabetic ketoacidosis. In patients with known diabetes, precipitating factors include infection, noncompliance with insulin, myocardial infarction, and gastrointestinal bleeding.
   B. **Symptoms of DKA** include polyuria, polydipsia, fatigue, nausea, and vomiting, developing over 1 to 2 days. Abdominal pain is prominent in 25%.
   C. **Physical examination**
      1. Patients are typically flushed, tachycardic, tachypneic, and volume depleted with dry mucous membranes. Kussmaul's respiration (rapid, deep breathing and air hunger) occurs when the serum pH is between 7.0 and 7.24.
      2. **A fruity odor** on the breath indicates the presence of acetone, a byproduct of diabetic ketoacidosis.
      3. **Fever**, although seldom present, indicates infection. Eighty percent of patients with diabetic ketoacidosis have altered mental status. Most are awake but confused; 10% are comatose.
   D. **Laboratory findings**
      1. Serum glucose level >300 mg/dL
      2. pH <7.35, pCO_2 <40 mm Hg
      3. Bicarbonate level below normal with an elevated anion gap
      4. Presence of ketones in the serum
II. **Differential diagnosis**
   A. **Differential diagnosis of ketosis-causing conditions**
      1. **Alcoholic ketoacidosis** occurs with heavy drinking and vomiting. It does not cause an elevated glucose.
      2. **Starvation ketosis** occurs after 24 hours without food and is not usually confused with DKA because glucose and serum pH are normal.
   B. **Differential diagnosis of acidosis-causing conditions**
      1. **Metabolic acidoses** are divided into increased anion gap (>14 mEq/L) and normal anion gap; anion gap = sodium - (Cl^- + HCO_3^-).
      2. **Anion gap acidoses** can be caused by ketoacidoses, lactic acidosis, uremia, salicylate, methanol, ethanol, or ethylene glycol poisoning.
      3. **Non-anion gap acidoses** are associated with a normal glucose level and absent serum ketones. Causes of non-anion gap acidoses include renal or gastrointestinal bicarbonate loss.
   C. **Hyperglycemia caused by hyperosmolar nonketotic coma** occurs in patients with type 2 diabetes with severe hyperglycemia. Patients are

usually elderly and have a precipitating illness. Glucose level is markedly elevated (>600 mg/dL), osmolarity is increased, and ketosis is minimal.

III. Treatment of diabetic ketoacidosis

A. Fluid resuscitation

1. Fluid deficits average 5 liters or 50 mL/kg. Resuscitation consists of 1 liter of normal saline over the first hour and a second liter over the second and third hours. Thereafter, 1/2 normal saline should be infused at 100-120 mL/hr.

2. When the glucose level decreases to 250 mg/dL, 5% dextrose should be added to the replacement fluids to prevent hypoglycemia. If the glucose level declines rapidly, 10% dextrose should be infused along with regular insulin until the anion gap normalizes.

B. Insulin

1. An initial loading dose consists of 0.1 U/kg IV bolus. Insulin is then infused at 0.1 U/kg per hour. The biologic half-life of IV insulin is less than 20 minutes. The insulin infusion should be adjusted each hour so that the glucose decline does not exceed 100 mg/dL per hour.

2. The insulin infusion rate may be decreased when the bicarbonate level is greater than 20 mEq/L, the anion gap is less than 16 mEq/L, or the glucose is <250 mg/dL.

C. Potassium

1. The most common preventable cause of death in patients with DKA is hypokalemia. The typical deficit is between 300 and 500 mEq.

2. Potassium chloride should be started when fluid therapy is started. In most patients, the initial rate of potassium replacement is 20 mEq/h, but hypokalemia requires more aggressive replacement (40 mEq/h).

3. All patients should receive potassium replacement, except for those with renal failure, no urine output, or an initial serum potassium level greater than 6.0 mEq/L.

D. Sodium. For every 100 mg/dL that glucose is elevated, the sodium level should be assumed to be higher than the measured value by 1.6 mEq/L.

E. Phosphate. Diabetic ketoacidosis depletes phosphate stores. Serum phosphate level should be checked after 4 hours of treatment. If it is below 1.5 mg/dL, potassium phosphate should be added to the IV solution in place of KCl.

F. Bicarbonate therapy is not required unless the arterial pH value is <7.0. For a pH of <7.0, add 50 mEq of sodium bicarbonate to the first liter of IV fluid.

G. Magnesium. The usual magnesium deficit is 2-3 gm. If the patient's magnesium level is less than 1.8 mEq/L or if tetany is present, magnesium sulfate is given as 5g in 500 mL of 0.45% normal saline over 5 hours.

H. Additional therapies

1. A nasogastric tube should be inserted in semiconscious patients to protect against aspiration.

2. Deep vein thrombosis prophylaxis with subcutaneous heparin should be provided for patients who are elderly, unconscious, or severely hyperosmolar (5,000 U every 12 hours).

IV. Monitoring of therapy

A. Serum bicarbonate level and anion gap should be monitored to determine the effectiveness of insulin therapy.

B. Glucose levels should be checked at 1-2 hour intervals during IV insulin administration.

C. Electrolyte levels should be assessed every 2 hours for the first 6-8

hours, and then q8h. Phosphorus and magnesium levels should be checked after 4 hours of treatment.

D. Plasma and urine ketones are helpful in diagnosing diabetic ketoacidosis, but are not necessary during therapy.

V. Determining the underlying cause

A. Infection is the underlying cause of diabetic ketoacidosis in 50% of cases. Infection of the urinary tract, respiratory tract, skin, sinuses, ears, or teeth should be sought. Fever is unusual in diabetic ketoacidosis and indicates infection when present. If infection is suspected, antibiotics should be promptly initiated.

B. Omission of insulin doses is often a precipitating factor. Myocardial infarction, ischemic stroke, and abdominal catastrophes may precipitate DKA.

VI. Initiation of subcutaneous insulin

A. When the serum bicarbonate and anion gap levels are normal, subcutaneous regular insulin can be started.

B. Intravenous and subcutaneous administration of insulin should overlap to avoid redevelopment of ketoacidosis. The intravenous infusion may be stopped 1 hour after the first subcutaneous injection of insulin.

C. Estimation of subcutaneous insulin requirements

1. Multiply the final insulin infusion rate times 24 hours. Two-thirds of the total dose is given in the morning as two-thirds NPH and one-third regular insulin. The remaining one-third of the total dose is given before supper as one-half NPH and one-half regular insulin.

2. Subsequent doses should be adjusted according to the patient's blood glucose response.

Acute Renal Failure

Acute renal failure is defined as a sudden decrease in renal function sufficient to increase the concentration of nitrogenous wastes in the blood. It is characterized by an increasing BUN and creatinine.

I. Clinical presentation of acute renal failure

A. Oliguria is a common indicator of acute renal failure, and it is marked by a decrease in urine output to less than 30 mL/h. Acute renal failure may be oliguric (<500 L/day) or nonoliguric (>30 mL/h). Anuria (<100 mL/day) does not usually occur in renal failure, and its presence suggests obstruction or a vascular cause.

B. Acute renal failure may also be manifest by encephalopathy, volume overload, pericarditis, bleeding, anemia, hyperkalemia, hyperphosphatemia, hypocalcemia, and metabolic acidemia.

II. Clinical causes of renal failure

A. Prerenal insult

1. Prerenal insult is the most common cause of acute renal failure, accounting for 70% of cases. Prerenal failure is usually caused by reduced renal perfusion secondary to extracellular fluid loss (diarrhea, diuresis, GI hemorrhage) or secondary to extracellular fluid sequestration (pancreatitis, sepsis), inadequate cardiac output, renal vasoconstriction (sepsis, liver disease, drugs), or inadequate fluid intake or replacement.

2. Most patients with prerenal azotemia have oliguria, a history of large

fluid losses (vomiting, diarrhea, burns), and evidence of intravascular volume depletion (thirst, weight loss, orthostatic hypotension, tachycardia, flat neck veins, dry mucous membranes). Patients with congestive heart failure may have total body volume excess (distended neck veins, pulmonary and pedal edema) but still have compromised renal perfusion and prerenal azotemia because of diminished cardiac output.

3. Causes of prerenal failure are usually reversible if recognized and treated early; otherwise, prolonged renal hypoperfusion can lead to acute tubular necrosis and permanent renal insufficiency.

B. **Intrarenal insult**
   1. **Acute tubular necrosis (ATN)** is the most common intrinsic renal disease leading to ARF.
      a. **Prolonged renal hypoperfusion** is the most common cause of ATN.
      b. **Nephrotoxic agents** (aminoglycosides, heavy metals, radiocontrast media, ethylene glycol) represent exogenous nephrotoxins. ATN may also occur as a result of endogenous nephrotoxins, such as intratubular pigments (hemoglobinuria), intratubular proteins (myeloma), and intratubular crystals (uric acid).
   2. **Acute interstitial nephritis (AIN)** is an allergic reaction secondary to drugs (NSAIDs, β-lactams).
   3. **Arteriolar injury** occurs secondary to hypertension, vasculitis, microangiopathic disorders.
   4. **Glomerulonephritis** secondary to immunologically mediated inflammation may cause intrarenal damage.

C. **Postrenal insult** results from obstruction of urine flow. Postrenal insult is the least common cause of acute renal failure, accounting for 10%. Postrenal insult may be caused by obstruction secondary to prostate cancer, benign prostatic hypertrophy, or renal calculi. Postrenal insult may be caused by amyloidosis, uric acid crystals, multiple myeloma, methotrexate, or acyclovir.

III. **Clinical evaluation of acute renal failure**
   A. **Initial evaluation** of renal failure should determine whether the cause is decreased renal perfusion, obstructed urine flow, or disorders of the renal parenchyma. Volume status (orthostatic pulse, blood pressure, fluid intake and output, daily weights, hemodynamic parameters), nephrotoxic medications, and pattern of urine output should be assessed.
   B. **Prerenal azotemia** is likely when there is a history of heart failure or extracellular fluid volume loss or depletion.
   C. **Postrenal azotemia** is suggested by a history of decreased size or force of the urine stream, anuria, flank pain, hematuria or pyuria, or cancer of the bladder, prostate or pelvis.
   D. **Intrarenal insult** is suggested by a history of prolonged volume depletion (often post-surgical), pigmenturia, hemolysis, rhabdomyolysis, or nephrotoxins. Intrarenal insult is suggested by recent radiocontrast, aminoglycoside use, or vascular catheterization. Interstitial nephritis may be implicated by a history of medication rash, fever, or arthralgias.
   E. **Chronic renal failure** is suggested by diabetes mellitus, normochromic normocytic anemia, hypercalcemia, and hyperphosphatemia.

IV. **Physical examination**
   A. Cardiac output, volume status, bladder size, and systemic disease manifestations should be assessed.
   B. **Prerenal azotemia** is suggested by impaired cardiac output (neck vein

distention, pulmonary rales, pedal edema). Volume depletion is suggested by orthostatic blood pressure changes, weight loss, low urine output, or diuretic use.

  C. **Flank, suprapubic, or abdominal masses** may indicate an obstructive cause.

  D. **Skin rash** suggests drug-induced interstitial nephritis; palpable purpura suggests vasculitis; nonpalpable purpura suggests thrombotic thrombo cytopenic purpura or hemolytic-uremic syndrome.

  E. **Bladder catheterization** is useful to rule out suspected bladder outlet obstruction. A residual volume of more than 100 mL suggests bladder outlet obstruction.

  F. **Central venous monitoring** is used to measure cardiac output and left ventricular filling pressure if prerenal failure is suspected.

V. **Laboratory evaluation**

  A. **Spot urine sodium concentration**

    1. Spot urine sodium can help distinguish between prerenal azotemia and acute tubular necrosis.

    2. Prerenal failure causes increased reabsorption of salt and water and will manifest as a low spot urine sodium concentration <20 mEq/L and a low fractional sodium excretion <1%, and a urine/plasma creatinine ration of >40. Fractional excretion of sodium (%) = ([urine sodium/plasma sodium] ÷ [urine creatinine/plasma creatinine] x 100).

    3. If tubular necrosis is the cause, the spot urine concentration will be >40 mEq/L, and fractional excretion of sodium will be >1%.

  B. **Urinalysis**

    1. **Normal urine sediment** is a strong indicator of prerenal azotemia or may be an indicator of obstructive uropathy.

    2. **Hematuria, pyuria, or crystals** may be associated with postrenal obstructive azotemia.

    3. **Abundant cells, casts, or protein** suggests an intrarenal disorder.

    4. **Red cells** alone may indicate vascular disorders. RBC casts and abundant protein suggest glomerular disease (glomerulonephritis).

    5. **White cell casts and eosinophilic casts** indicate interstitial nephritis.

    6. **Renal epithelial cell casts and pigmented granular casts** are associated with acute tubular necrosis.

  C. **Ultrasound** is useful for evaluation of suspected postrenal obstruction (nephrolithiasis). The presence of small (<10 cm in length), scarred kidneys is diagnostic of chronic renal insufficiency.

VI. **Management of acute renal failure**

  A. Reversible disorders, such as obstruction, should be excluded, and hypovolemia should be corrected with volume replacement. Cardiac output should be maintained. In critically ill patients, a pulmonary artery catheter should be used for evaluation and monitoring.

  B. **Extracellular fluid volume expansion.** Infusion of a 1-2 liter crystalloid fluid bolus may confirm suspected volume depletion.

  C. If the patient remains oliguric despite euvolemia, IV diuretics may be administered. A large single dose of furosemide (100-200 mg) may be administered intravenously to promote diuresis. If urine flow is not improved, the dose of furosemide may be doubled. Furosemide may be repeated in 2 hours, or a continuous IV infusion of 10-40 mg/hr (max 1000 mg/day) may be used.

  D. The dosage or dosing intervals of renally excreted drugs should be modified.

    E. **Hyperkalemia** is the most immediately life-threatening complication of renal failure. Serum potassium values greater than 6.5 mEq/L may lead to arrhythmias and cardiac arrest. Potassium should be removed from IV solutions. Hyperkalemia may be treated with sodium polystyrene sulfonate (Kayexalate), 30-60 gm PO/PR every 4-6 hours.

    F. **Hyperphosphatemia** can be controlled with aluminum hydroxide antacids (eg, Amphojel or Basaljel), 15-30 ml or one to three capsules PO with meals, should be used.

    G. **Fluids.** After normal volume has been restored, fluid intake should be reduced to an amount equal to urinary and other losses plus insensible losses of 300-500 mL/day. In oliguric patients, daily fluid intake may need to be restricted to less than 1 L.

    H. **Nutritional therapy.** A renal diet consisting of daily high biologic value protein intake of 0.5 gm/kg/d, sodium 2 g, potassium 40-60 mg/day, and at least 35 kcal/kg of nonprotein calories is recommended. Phosphorus should be restricted to 800 mg/day

    I. **Dialysis.** Indications for dialysis include uremic pericarditis, severe hyperkalemia, pulmonary edema, persistent severe metabolic acidosis (pH less than 7.2), and symptomatic uremia.

Hyperkalemia

Body potassium is 98% intracellular. Only 2% of total body potassium, about 70 mEq, is in the extracellular fluid, with the normal concentration of 3.5-5 mEq/L.

I. **Pathophysiology of potassium homeostasis**
    A. The normal upper limit of plasma K is 5-5.5 mEq/L, with a mean K level of 4.3.

    B. **External potassium balance.** Normal dietary K intake is 1-1.5 mEq/kg in the form of vegetables and meats. The kidney is the primary organ for preserving external K balance, excreting 90% of the daily K burden.

    C. **Internal potassium balance.** Potassium transfer to and from tissues, is affected by insulin, acid-base status, catecholamines, aldosterone, plasma osmolality, cellular necrosis, and glucagon.

II. **Clinical disorders of external potassium balance**
    A. **Chronic renal failure.** The kidney is able to excrete the dietary intake of potassium until the glomerular filtration rate falls below 10 cc/minute or until urine output falls below 1 L/day. Renal failure is advanced before hyperkalemia occurs.

    B. **Impaired renal tubular function.** Renal diseases may cause hyperkalemia, and the renal tubular acidosis caused by these conditions may worsen hyperkalemia.

    C. **Primary adrenal insufficiency (Addison's disease)** is now a rare cause of hyperkalemia. Diagnosis is indicated by the combination of hyperkalemia and hyponatremia and is confirmed by a low aldosterone and a low plasma cortisol level that does not respond to adrenocorticotropic hormone treatment.

    D. **Drugs** that may cause hyperkalemia include nonsteroidal anti-inflammatory drugs, angiotensin-converting enzyme inhibitors, cyclosporine, and potassium-sparing diuretics. Hyperkalemia is especially common when these drugs are given to patients at risk for hyperkalemia (diabetics, renal failure, advanced age).

E. **Excessive potassium intake**
  1. Long-term potassium supplementation results in hyperkalemia most often when an underlying impairment in renal excretion already exists.
  2. Intravenous administration of 0.5 mEq/kg over 1 hour increases serum levels by 0.6 mEq/L. Hyperkalemia often results when infusions of greater than 40 mEq/hour are given.

III. **Clinical disorders of internal potassium balance**
  A. **Diabetic patients** are at particular risk for severe hyperkalemia because of renal insufficiency and hyporeninemic hypoaldosteronism.
  B. **Systemic acidosis** reduces renal excretion of potassium and moves potassium out of cells, resulting in hyperkalemia.
  C. **Endogenous potassium release** from muscle injury, tumor lysis, or chemotherapy may elevate serum potassium.

IV. **Manifestations of hyperkalemia**
  A. Hyperkalemia, unless severe, is usually asymptomatic. The effect of hyperkalemia on the heart becomes significant above 6 mEq/L. As levels increase, the initial ECG change is tall peaked T waves. The QT interval is normal or diminished.
  B. As K levels rise further, the PR interval becomes prolonged, then the P wave amplitude decreases. The QRS complex eventually widens into a sine wave pattern, with subsequent cardiac standstill.
  C. At serum K is >7 mEq/L, muscle weakness may lead to a flaccid paralysis. Sensory abnormalities, impaired speech and respiratory arrest may follow.

V. **Pseudohyperkalemia**
  A. Potassium may be falsely elevated by hemolysis during phlebotomy, when K is released from ischemic muscle distal to a tourniquet, and because of erythrocyte fragility disorders.
  B. Falsely high laboratory measurement of serum potassium may occur with markedly elevated platelet counts (>10^6 platelet/mm^3) or white blood cell counts (>50,000/mm^3).

VI. **Diagnostic approach to hyperkalemia**
  A. The serum K level should be repeat tested to rule out laboratory error. If significant thrombocytosis or leukocytosis is present, a plasma potassium level should be determined.
  B. The 24-hour urine output, urinary K excretion, blood urea nitrogen, and serum creatinine should be measured. Renal K retention is diagnosed when urinary K excretion is less than 20 mEq/day.
  C. High urinary K, excretion of >20 mEq/day, is indicative of excessive K intake as the cause.

VII. **Renal hyperkalemia**
  A. If urinary K excretion is low and urine output is in the oliguric range, and creatinine clearance is lower than 20 cc/minute, renal failure is the probable cause. Prerenal azotemia resulting from volume depletion must be ruled out because the hyperkalemia will respond to volume restoration.
  B. When urinary K excretion is low, yet blood urea nitrogen and creatinine levels are not elevated and urine volume is at least 1 L daily and renal sodium excretion is adequate (about 20 mEq/day), then either a defect in the secretion of renin or aldosterone or tubular resistance to aldosterone is likely. Low plasma renin and aldosterone levels, will confirm the diagnosis of hyporeninemic hypoaldosteronism. Addison's disease is suggested by a low serum cortisol, and the diagnosis is confirmed with a ACTH (Cortrosyn) stimulation test.
  C. When inadequate K excretion is not caused by hypoaldosteronism, a

tubular defect in K clearance is suggested. Urinary tract obstruction, renal transplant, lupus, or a medication should be considered.

VIII. Extrarenal hyperkalemia
   A. When hyperkalemia occurs along with high urinary K excretion of >20 mEq/day, excessive intake of K is the cause. Potassium excess in IV fluids, diet, or medication should be sought. A concomitant underlying renal defect in K excretion is also likely to be present.
   B. Blood sugar should be measured to rule out insulin deficiency; blood pH and serum bicarbonate should be measured to rule out acidosis.
   C. Endogenous sources of K, such as tissue necrosis, hypercatabolism, hematoma, gastrointestinal bleeding, or intravascular hemolysis should be excluded.

IX. Management of hyperkalemia
   A. Acute treatment of hyperkalemia
      1. Calcium
         a. If the electrocardiogram shows loss of P waves or widening of QRS complexes, calcium should be given IV; calcium reduces the cell membrane threshold potential.
         b. Calcium chloride (10%) 2-3 g should be given over 5 minutes. In patients with circulatory compromise, 1 g of calcium chloride IV should be given over 3 minutes.
         c. If the serum K level is greater than 7 mEq/L, calcium should be given. If digitalis intoxication is suspected, calcium must be given cautiously. Coexisting hyponatremia should be treated with hypertonic saline.
      2. Insulin: If the only ECG abnormalities are peaked T waves and the serum level is under 7 mEq/L, treatment should begin with insulin (regular insulin, 5-10 U by IV push) with 50% dextrose water (D50W) 50 mL IV push. Repeated insulin doses of 10 U and glucose can be given every 15 minutes for maximal effect.
      3. Sodium bicarbonate promotes cellular uptake of K. It should be given as 1-2 vials (50-mEq/vials) IV push.
      4. Potassium elimination measures
         a. Sodium polystyrene sulfonate (Kayexalate) is a cation exchange resin which binds to potassium in the lower GI tract. Dosage is 30-60 gm premixed with sorbitol 20% PO/PR.
         b. Furosemide (Lasix) 100 mg IV should be given to promote kaliuresis.
         c. Emergent hemodialysis for hyperkalemia is rarely necessary except when refractory metabolic acidosis is present.

Hypokalemia

Hypokalemia is characterized by a serum potassium concentration of less than 3.5 mEq/L. Ninety-eight percent of K is intracellular.

I. Pathophysiology of hypokalemia
   A. Cellular redistribution of potassium. Hypokalemia may result from the intracellular shift of potassium by insulin, beta-2 agonist drugs, stress induced catecholamine release, thyrotoxic periodic paralysis, and alkalosis-induced shift (metabolic or respiratory).
   B. Nonrenal potassium loss
      1. Gastrointestinal loss can be caused by diarrhea, laxative abuse, villous adenoma, biliary drainage, enteric fistula, clay ingestion, potassium

binding resin ingestion, or nasogastric suction.
2. Sweating, prolonged low-potassium diet, hemodialysis and peritoneal dialysis may also cause nonrenal potassium loss.

C. **Renal potassium loss**
1. **Hypertensive high renin states.** Malignant hypertension, renal artery stenosis, renin-producing tumors.
2. **Hypertensive low renin, high aldosterone states.** Primary hyperaldosteronism (adenoma or hyperplasia).
3. **Hypertensive low renin, low aldosterone states.** Congenital adrenal hyperplasia (11 or 17 hydroxylase deficiency), Cushing's syndrome or disease, exogenous mineralocorticoids (Florinef, licorice, chewing tobacco), Liddle's syndrome.
4. **Normotensive states**
   a. **Metabolic acidosis.** Renal tubular acidosis (type I or II)
   b. **Metabolic alkalosis (urine chloride <10 mEq/day).** Vomiting
   c. **Metabolic alkalosis (urine chloride >10 mEq/day).** Bartter's syndrome, diuretics, magnesium depletion, normotensive hyperaldosteronism
5. **Drugs** associated with potassium loss include amphotericin B, ticarcillin, piperacillin, and loop diuretics.

II. **Clinical effects of hypokalemia**
A. **Cardiac effects**. The most lethal consequence of hypokalemia is cardiac arrhythmia. Electrocardiographic effects include a depressed ST segment, decreased T-wave amplitude, U waves, and a prolonged QT-U interval.
B. **Musculoskeletal effects.** The initial manifestation of K depletion is muscle weakness, which can lead to paralysis. In severe cases, respiratory muscle paralysis may occur.
C. **Gastrointestinal effects.** Nausea, vomiting, constipation, and paralytic ileus may develop.

III. **Diagnostic evaluation**
A. The 24-hour urinary potassium excretion should be measured. If >20 mEq/day, excessive urinary K loss is the cause. If <20 mEq/d, low K intake, or non-urinary K loss is the cause.
B. In patients with excessive renal K loss and hypertension, plasma renin and aldosterone should be measured to differentiate adrenal from non-adrenal causes of hyperaldosteronism.
C. If hypertension is absent and serum pH is acidotic, renal tubular acidosis should be considered. If hypertension is absent and serum pH is normal to alkalotic, a high urine chloride (>10 mEq/d) suggests hypokalemia secondary to diuretics or Bartter's syndrome. A low urine chloride (<10 mEq/d) suggests vomiting.

IV. **Emergency treatment of hypokalemia**
A. **Indications for urgent replacement.** Electrocardiographic abnormalities, myocardial infarction, hypoxia, digitalis intoxication, marked muscle weakness, or respiratory muscle paralysis.
B. **Intravenous potassium therapy**
1. Intravenous KCL is usually used unless concomitant hypophosphatemia is present, where potassium phosphate is indicated.
2. The maximal rate of intravenous K replacement is 30 mEq/hour. The K concentration of IV fluids should be 80 mEq/L or less if given via a peripheral vein. Frequent monitoring of serum K and constant electrocardiographic monitoring is recommended when potassium levels are being replaced.

V. Non-emergent treatment of hypokalemia
A. Attempts should be made to normalize K levels if <3.5 mEq/L.
B. Oral supplementation is significantly safer than IV. Liquid formulations are preferred due to rapid oral absorption, compared to sustained release formulations, which are absorbed over several hours.
1. KCL elixir 20-40 mEq qd-tid PO after meals.
2. Micro-K, 10 mEq tabs, 2-3 tabs tid PO after meals (40-100 mEq/d).

Hypomagnesemia

Magnesium deficiency occurs in up to 11% of hospitalized patients. The normal range of serum magnesium is 1.5 to 2.0 mEq/L, which is maintained by the kidney, intestine, and bone.

I. Pathophysiology
A. **Decreased magnesium intake.** Protein-calorie malnutrition, prolonged parenteral fluid administration, and catabolic illness are common causes of hypomagnesemia.
B. **Gastrointestinal losses of magnesium** may result from prolonged nasogastric suction, laxative abuse, and pancreatitis.
C. **Renal losses of magnesium**
1. Renal loss of magnesium may occur secondary to renal tubular acidosis, glomerulonephritis, interstitial nephritis, or acute tubular necrosis.
2. Hyperthyroidism, hypercalcemia, and hypophosphatemia may cause magnesium loss.
3. **Agents that enhance renal magnesium excretion** include alcohol, loop and thiazide diuretics, amphotericin B, aminoglycosides, cisplatin, and pentamidine.
D. **Alterations in magnesium distribution**
1. Redistribution of circulating magnesium occurs by extracellular to intracellular shifts, sequestration, hungry bone syndrome, or by acute administration of glucose, insulin, or amino acids.
2. Magnesium depletion can be caused by large quantities of parenteral fluids and pancreatitis-induced sequestration of magnesium.

II. Clinical manifestations of hypomagnesemia
A. **Neuromuscular findings** may include positive Chvostek's and Trousseau's signs, tremors, myoclonic jerks, seizures, and coma.
B. **Cardiovascular.** Ventricular tachycardia, ventricular fibrillation, atrial fibrillation, multifocal atrial tachycardia, ventricular ectopic beats, hypertension, enhancement of digoxin-induced dysrhythmias, and cardiomyopathies.
C. **ECG changes** include ventricular arrhythmias (extrasystoles, tachycardia) and atrial arrhythmias (atrial fibrillation, supraventricular tachycardia, torsades de Pointes). Prolonged PR and QT intervals, ST segment depression, T-wave inversions, wide QRS complexes, and tall T-waves may occur.

III. Clinical evaluation
A. Hypomagnesemia is diagnosed when the serum magnesium is less than 0.7-0.8 mmol/L. Symptoms of magnesium deficiency occur when the serum magnesium concentration is less than 0.5 mmol/L. A 24-hour urine collection for magnesium is the first step in the evaluation of hypomagnesemia. Hypomagnesia caused by renal magnesium loss is

associated with magnesium excretion that exceeds 24 mg/day.
  B. Low urinary magnesium excretion (<1 mmol/day), with concomitant serum hypomagnesemia, suggests magnesium deficiency due to decreased intake, nonrenal losses, or redistribution of magnesium.
IV. **Treatment of hypomagnesemia**
  A. **Asymptomatic magnesium deficiency**
    1. In hospitalized patients, the daily magnesium requirements can be provided through either a balanced diet, as oral magnesium supplements (0.36-0.46 mEq/kg/day), or 16-30 mEq/day in a parenteral nutrition formulation.
    2. Magnesium oxide is better absorbed and less likely to cause diarrhea than magnesium sulfate. Magnesium oxide preparations include Mag-Ox 400 (240 mg elemental magnesium per 400 mg tablet), Uro-Mag (84 mg elemental magnesium per 400 mg tablet), and magnesium chloride (Slo-Mag) 64 mg/tab, 1-2 tabs bid.
  B. **Symptomatic magnesium deficiency**
    1. Serum magnesium $\leq$0.5 mmol/L requires IV magnesium repletion with electrocardiographic and respiratory monitoring.
    2. Magnesium sulfate 1-6 gm in 500 mL of D5W can be infused IV at 1 gm/hr. An additional 6-9 gm of $MgSO_4$ should be given by continuous infusion over the next 24 hours.

Hypermagnesemia

Serum magnesium has a normal range of 0.8-1.2 mmol/L. Magnesium homeostasis is regulated by renal and gastrointestinal mechanisms. Hypermagnesemia is usually iatrogenic and is frequently seen in conjunction with renal insufficiency.

I. **Clinical evaluation of hypermagnesemia**
  A. **Causes of hypermagnesemia**
    1. **Renal.** Creatinine clearance <30 mL/minute.
    2. **Nonrenal.** Excessive use of magnesium cathartics, especially with renal failure; iatrogenic overtreatment with magnesium sulfate.
  B. **Cardiovascular manifestations of hypermagnesemia**
    1. **Hypermagnesemia <10 mEq/L.** Delayed interventricular conduction, first-degree heart block, prolongation of the Q-T interval.
    2. **Levels greater than 10 mEq/L.** Low-grade heart block progressing to complete heart block and asystole occurs at levels greater than 12.5 mmol/L (>6.25 mmol/L).
  C. **Neuromuscular effects**
    1. Hyporeflexia occurs at a magnesium level >4 mEq/L (>2 mmol/L); diminution of deep tendon reflexes is an early sign of magnesium toxicity.
    2. Respiratory depression due to respiratory muscle paralysis, somnolence and coma occur at levels >13 mEq/L (6.5 mmol/L).
    3. Hypermagnesemia should always be considered when these symptoms occur in patients with renal failure, in those receiving therapeutic magnesium, and in laxative abuse.
II. **Treatment of hypermagnesemia**
  A. **Asymptomatic, hemodynamically stable patients**. Moderate hypermagnesemia can be managed by elimination of intake.

B. Severe hypermagnesemia
1. Furosemide 20-40 mg IV q3-4h should be given as needed. Saline diuresis should be initiated with 0.9% saline, infused at 120 cc/h to replace urine loss.
2. If ECG abnormalities (peaked T waves, loss of P waves, or widened QRS complexes) or if respiratory depression is present, IV calcium gluconate should be given as 1-3 ampules (10% solution, 1 gm per 10 mL amp), added to saline infusate. Calcium gluconate can be infused to reverse acute cardiovascular toxicity or respiratory failure as 15 mg/kg over a 4-hour period.
3. Parenteral insulin and glucose can be given to shift magnesium into cells. Dialysis is necessary for patients who have severe hypermagnesemia.

Disorders of Water and Sodium Balance

I. Pathophysiology of water and sodium balance
  A. Volitional intake of water is regulated by thirst. Maintenance intake of water is the amount of water sufficient to offset obligatory losses.
  B. Maintenance water needs
    = 100 mL/kg for first 10 kg of body weight
    + 50 mL/kg for next 10 kg
    + 20 mL/kg for weight greater than 20 kg
  C. Clinical signs of hyponatremia. Confusion, agitation, lethargy, seizures, and coma.
  D. Pseudohyponatremia
    1. Elevation of blood glucose may creates an osmotic gradient that pulls water from cells into the extracellular fluid, diluting the extracellular sodium. The contribution of hyperglycemia to hyponatremia can be estimated using the following formula:
    Expected change in serum sodium = (serum glucose - 100) x 0.016
    2. Marked elevation of plasma lipids or protein can also result in erroneous hyponatremia because of laboratory inaccuracy. The percentage of plasma water can be estimated with the following formula:
    % plasma water = 100 - [0.01 x lipids (mg/dL)] - [0.73 x protein (g/dL)]

II. Diagnostic evaluation of hyponatremia
  A. Pseudohyponatremia should be excluded by repeat testing. The cause of the hyponatremia should be determined based on history, physical exam, urine osmolality, serum osmolality, urine sodium and chloride. An assessment of volume status should determine if the patient is volume contracted, normal volume, or volume expanded.
  B. Classification of hyponatremic patients based on urine osmolality
    1. **Low-urine osmolality (50-180 mOsm/L)** indicates primary excessive water intake (psychogenic water drinking).
    2. **High-urine osmolality (urine osmolality >serum osmolality)**
      a. **High-urine sodium (>40 mEq/L) and volume contraction** indicates a renal source of sodium loss and fluid loss (excessive diuretic use, salt-wasting nephropathy, Addison's disease, osmotic diuresis).
      b. **High-urine sodium (>40 mEq/L) and normal volume** is most likely caused by water retention due to a drug effect, hypothyroidism, or the syndrome of inappropriate antidiuretic hormone secretion. In

SIADH, the urine sodium level is usually high. SIADH is found in the presence of a malignant tumor or a disorder of the pulmonary or central nervous system.

c. **Low-urine sodium (<20 mEq/L) and volume contraction,** dry mucous membranes, decreased skin turgor, and orthostatic hypotension indicate an extrarenal source of fluid loss (gastrointestinal disease, burns).

d. **Low-urine sodium (<20 mEq/L) and volume-expansion, and edema** is caused by congestive heart failure, cirrhosis with ascites, or nephrotic syndrome. Effective arterial blood volume is decreased. Decreased renal perfusion causes increased reabsorption of water.

Drugs Associated with SIADH

Acetaminophen	Isoproterenol
Barbiturates	Prostaglandin E$_1$
Carbamazepine	Meperidine
Chlorpropamide	Nicotine
Clofibrate	Tolbutamide
Cyclophosphamide	Vincristine
Indomethacin	

III. Treatment of water excess hyponatremia

A. Determine the volume of water excess

Water excess = total body water x ([140/measured sodium] -1)

B. Treatment of asymptomatic hyponatremia.
Water intake should be restricted to 1,000 mL/day. Food alone in the diet contains this much water, so no liquids should be consumed. If an intravenous solution is needed, an isotonic solution of 0.9% sodium chloride (normal saline) should be used. Dextrose should not be used in the infusion because the dextrose is metabolized into water.

C. Treatment of symptomatic hyponatremia

1. If neurologic symptoms of hyponatremia are present, the serum sodium level should be corrected with hypertonic saline. Excessively rapid correction of sodium may result in a syndrome of central pontine demyelination.

2. The serum sodium should be raised at a rate of 1 mEq/L per hour. If hyponatremia has been chronic, the rate should be limited to 0.5 mEq/L per hour. The goal of initial therapy is a serum sodium of 125-130 mEq/L, then water restriction should be continued until the level normalizes.

3. The amount of hypertonic saline needed is estimated using the following formula:
Sodium needed (mEq) = 0.6 x wt in kg x (desired sodium - measured sodium)

4. Hypertonic 3% sodium chloride contains 513 mEq/L of sodium. The calculated volume required should be administered over the period required to raise the serum sodium level at a rate of 0.5-1 mEq/L per hour. Concomitant administration of furosemide may be required to lessen the risk of fluid overload.

IV. Hypernatremia

A. Clinical manifestations of hypernatremia:
Clinical manifestations include tremulousness, irritability, ataxia, spasticity, mental confusion, seizures, and coma.

B. Causes of hypernatremia

1. Net sodium gain or net water loss will cause hypernatremia
2. Failure to replace obligate water losses may cause hypernatremia, as in patients unable to obtain water because of an altered mental status or severe debilitating disease.
3. **Diabetes insipidus:** If urine volume is high but urine osmolality is low, diabetes insipidus is the most likely cause.

Drugs Associated with Diabetes Insipidus	
Ethanol	Glyburide
Phenytoin	Amphotericin B
Chlorpromazine	Colchicine
Lithium	Vinblastine

C. Diagnosis of hypernatremia

1. Assessment of urine volume and osmolality are essential in the evaluation of hyperosmolality. The usual renal response to hypernatremia is the excretion of the minimum volume ($\leq$500 mL/day) of maximally concentrated urine (urine osmolality >800 mOsm/kg). These findings suggest extrarenal water loss.
2. Diabetes insipidus generally presents with polyuria and hypotonic urine (urine osmolality <250 mOsm/kg).

V. Management of hypernatremia

A. If there is evidence of hemodynamic compromise (eg, orthostatic hypotension, marked oliguria), fluid deficits should be corrected initially with isotonic saline. Once hemodynamic stability is achieved, the remaining free water deficit should be corrected with 5% dextrose water or 0.45% NaCl.

B. The water deficit can be estimated using the following formula:
Water deficit = 0.6 x wt in kg x (1 - [140/measured sodium]).

C. The change in sodium concentration should not exceed 1 mEq/liter/hour. One-half of the calculated water deficit can be administered in the first 24 hours, followed by correction of the remaining deficit over the next 1-2 days. The serum sodium concentration and ECF volume status should be evaluated every 6 hours. Excessively rapid correction of hypernatremia may lead to lethargy and seizures secondary to cerebral edema.

D. Maintenance fluid needs from ongoing renal and insensible losses must also be provided. If the patient is conscious and able to drink, water should be given orally or by nasogastric tube.

E. **Treatment of diabetes insipidus**

1. **Vasopressin (Pitressin)** 5-10 U IV/SQ q6h; fast onset of action with short duration.
2. **Desmopressin (DDAVP)** 2-4 mcg IV/SQ q12h; slow onset of action with long duration of effect.

VI. Mixed disorders

A. **Water excess and saline deficit** occurs when severe vomiting and diarrhea occur in a patient who is given only water. Clinical signs of volume contraction and a low serum sodium are present. Saline deficit is replaced and free water intake restricted until the serum sodium level has normalized.

B. **Water and saline excess** often occurs with heart failure, manifesting as edema and a low serum sodium. An increase in the extracellular fluid volume, as evidenced by edema, is a saline excess. A marked excess of free water expands the extracellular fluid volume, causing apparent hyponatremia. However, the important derangement in edema is an excess of sodium. Sodium and water restriction and use of furosemide are usually indicated in addition to treatment of the underlying disorder.

C. **Water and saline deficit** is frequently caused by vomiting and high fever and is characterized by signs of volume contraction and an elevated serum sodium. Saline and free water should be replaced in addition to maintenance amounts of water.

Hypercalcemic Crisis

Hypercalcemic crisis is defined as an elevation in serum calcium that is associated with volume depletion, mental status changes, and life-threatening cardiac arrhythmias. Hypercalcemic crisis is most commonly caused by malignancy-associated bone resorption.

I. **Diagnosis**
  A. Hypercalcemic crisis is often complicated by nausea, vomiting, hypovolemia, mental status changes, and hypotension.
  B. A correction for the low albumin level must be made because ionized calcium is the physiological important form of calcium.

  Corrected serum calcium (mg/dL) = serum calcium + 0.8 x (4.0 - albumin [g/dL])

  C. Most patients in hypercalcemic crisis have a corrected serum calcium level greater than 13 mg/dL.
  D. The ECG often demonstrates a short QT interval. Bradyarrhythmias, heart blocks, and cardiac arrest may also occur.

II. **Treatment of hypercalcemic crisis**
  A. Normal saline should be administered until the patient is normovolemic. If signs of fluid overload develop, furosemide (Lasix) can be given to promote sodium and calcium diuresis. Thiazide diuretics, vitamin D supplements and antacids containing sodium bicarbonate should be discontinued.
  B. Pamidronate disodium (Aredia) is the agent of choice for long-term treatment of hypercalcemia. A single dose of 90-mg infused IV over 24 hours should normalize calcium levels in 4 to 7 days. The pamidronate dose of 30- to 90-mg IV infusion may be repeated 7 days after the initial dose. Smaller doses (30 or 60 mg IV over 4 hours) are given every few weeks to maintain normal calcium levels.
  C. Calcitonin (Calcimar, Miacalcin) has the advantage of decreasing serum calcium levels within hours; 4 to 8 U/kg SQ/IM q12h. Calcitonin should be used in conjunction with pamidronate in severely hypercalcemic patients.

Hypophosphatemia

Clinical manifestations of hypophosphatemia include heart failure, muscle weakness, tremor, ataxia, seizures, coma, respiratory failure, delayed weaning from ventilator, hemolysis, and rhabdomyolysis.

I. Differential diagnosis of hypophosphatemia
   A. Increased urinary excretion: Hyperparathyroidism, renal tubular defects, diuretics.
   B. Decrease in GI absorption: Malnutrition, malabsorption, phosphate binding minerals (aluminum-containing antacids).
   C. Abnormal vitamin D metabolism: Vitamin D deficiency, familial hypophosphatemia, tumor-associated hypercalcemia.
   D. Intracellular shifts of phosphate: Diabetic ketoacidosis, respiratory alkalosis, alcohol withdrawal, recovery phase of starvation.

II. Labs: Phosphate, SMA 12, LDH, magnesium, calcium, albumin, PTH, urine electrolytes. 24-hr urine phosphate, and creatinine.

III. Diagnostic approach to hypophosphatemia
   A. 24-hr urine phosphate
   1. If 24-hour urine phosphate is less than 100 mg/day, the cause is gastrointestinal losses (emesis, diarrhea, NG suction, phosphate binders), vitamin D deficit, refeeding, recovery from burns, alkalosis, alcoholism, or DKA.
   2. If 24-hour urine phosphate is greater than 100 mg/day, the cause is renal losses, hyperparathyroidism, hypomagnesemia, hypokalemia, acidosis, diuresis, renal tubular defects, or vitamin D deficiency.

IV. Treatment
   A. Mild hypophosphatemia (1.0-2.5 mEq/dL)
   1. Na or K phosphate 0.25 mMol/kg IV infusion at the rate of 10 mMol/hr (in NS or D5W 150-250 mL), may repeat as needed.
   2. Neutral phosphate (Nutra-Phos), 2 packs PO bid-tid (250 mg elemental phosphorus/pack).

   B. Severe hypophosphatemia (<1.0 mEq/dL)
   1. Administer Na or K phosphate 0.5 m Moles/Kg IV infusion at the rate of 10 mMoles/hr (NS or D5W 150-250 mL), may repeat as needed.
   2. Add potassium phosphate to IV solution in place of KCl (max 80 mEq/L infused at 100-150 mL/h). Max IV dose 7.5 mg phosphorus/kg/6h **OR** 2.5-5 mg elemental phosphorus/kg IV over 6h. Give as potassium or sodium phosphate (93 mg phosphate/mL and 4 mEq Na+ or K+/mL). Do not mix calcium and phosphorus in same IV.

Hyperphosphatemia

I. Clinical manifestations of hyperphosphatemia: Hypotension, bradycardia, arrhythmias, bronchospasm, apnea, laryngeal spasm, tetany, seizures, weakness, psychosis, confusion.

II. Clinical evaluation of hyperphosphatemia
   A. Exogenous phosphate administration: Enemas, laxatives, diphosphonates, vitamin D excess.
   B. Endocrine disturbances: Hypoparathyroidism, acromegaly, PTH resistance.

    C. Labs: Phosphate, SMA 12, calcium, parathyroid hormone. 24-hr urine phosphate, creatinine.
III. Therapy: Correct hypocalcemia, restrict dietary phosphate, saline diuresis.
    A. Moderate hyperphosphatemia
        1. Aluminum hydroxide (Amphojel) 5-10 mL or 1-2 tablets PO ac tid; aluminum containing agents bind to intestinal phosphate, and decreases absorption **OR**
        2. Aluminum carbonate (Basaljel) 5-10 mL or 1-2 tablets PO ac tid **OR**
        3. Calcium carbonate (Oscal) (250 or 500 mg elemental calcium/tab) 1-2 gm elemental calcium PO ac tid. Keep calcium-phosphate product <70; start only if phosphate <5.5.
    B. Severe hyperphosphatemia
        1. Volume expansion with 0.9% saline 1 L over 1h if the patient is not azotemic.
        2. Dialysis is recommended for patients with renal failure.

References

References may be obtained at www.ccspublishing.com.

Commonly Used Formulas

A-a gradient = $[(P_B-PH_2O) FiO_2-PCO_2/R]-PO_2$ arterial

$\qquad\qquad = (713 \times FiO_2-pCO_2/0.8) -pO_2$ arterial

P_B = 760 mm Hg; PH_2O = 47 mm Hg; R ≈ 0.8
normal Aa gradient <10-15 mm Hg (room air)

Arterial O_2 content = 1.36(Hgb)(SaO_2)+0.003(PaO_2)

O_2 delivery = CO x arterial O_2 content

Cardiac output = HR x stroke volume
Normal CO = 4-6 L/min

$SVR = \dfrac{MAP-CVP}{CO_{L/min}} \times 80$ = NL 800-1200 dyne/sec/cm^2

$PVR = \dfrac{PA-PCWP}{CO_{L/min}} \times 80$ = NL 45-120 dyne/sec/cm^2

Normal creatinine clearance = 100-125 mL/min(males), 85-105(females)

Body water deficit (L) = $\dfrac{0.6(weight\ kg)([measured\ serum\ Na]-140)}{140}$

Osmolality mOsm/kg = 2[Na+ K] + $\dfrac{BUN}{2.8}$ + $\dfrac{glucose}{18}$ = NL 270-290 $\dfrac{mOsm}{kg}$

Fractional excreted Na = $\dfrac{U\ Na/\ Serum\ Na}{U\ Cr/\ Serum\ Cr} \times 100$ = NL<1%

Anion Gap = Na + K-(Cl + HCO_3)

For each 100 mg/dL ↑ in glucose, Na+ ↓ by 1.6 mEq/L.

Corrected serum Ca^+ (mg/dL) = measured Ca mg/dL + 0.8 x (4-albumin g/dL)

Basal energy expenditure (BEE):
  Males=66 + (13.7 x actual weight Kg) + (5 x height cm)-(6.8 x age)
  Females= 655+(9.6 x actual weight Kg)+(1.7 x height cm)-(4.7 x age)

Nitrogen Balance = Gm protein intake/6.25-urine urea nitrogen-(3-4 gm/d insensible loss)

Commonly Used Drug Levels

Drug	Therapeutic Range*
Amikacin	Peak 25-30; trough <10 mcg/mL
Amiodarone	1.0-3.0 mcg/mL
Amitriptyline	100-250 ng/mL
Carbamazepine	4-10 mcg/mL
Chloramphenicol	Peak 10-15; trough <5 mcg/mL
Desipramine	150-300 ng/mL
Digoxin	0.8-2.0 ng/mL
Disopyramide	2-5 mcg/mL
Doxepin	75-200 ng/mL
Flecainide	0.2-1.0 mcg/mL
Gentamicin	Peak 6.0-8.0; trough <2.0 mcg/mL

Imipramine .... 150-300 ng/mL
Lidocaine .... 2-5 mcg/mL
Lithium .... 0.5-1.4 mEq/L
Nortriptyline .... 50-150 ng/mL
Phenobarbital .... 10-30 mEq/mL
Phenytoin** .... 8-20 mcg/mL
Procainamide .... 4.0-8.0 mcg/mL
Quinidine .... 2.5-5.0 mcg/mL
Salicylate .... 15-25 mg/dL
Theophylline .... 8-20 mcg/mL
Valproic acid .... 50-100 mcg/mL
Vancomycin .... Peak 30-40; trough <10 mcg/mL

* The therapeutic range of some drugs may vary depending on the reference lab used.
** Therapeutic range of phenytoin is 4-10 mcg/mL in presence of significant azotemia and/or hypoalbuminemia.

Drugs that Prolong the QT-Interval

Amiodarone	Naratriptan
Bepridil	Nicardipine
Chlorpromazine	Octreotide
Desipramine	Pentamidine
Disopyramide	Pimozide
Dofetilide	Probucol
Droperidol	Procainamide
Erythromycin	Quetiapine
Flecainide	Quinidine
Fluoxetine	Risperidone
Foscarnet	salmeterol
Fosphenytoin	Sotalol
Gatifolixin	Sparfloxacin
Halofantrine	Sumatriptan
Haloperidol	Tamoxifen
Ibutilide	Thioridazine
Isradipine	Venlafaxine
Mesoridazine	Zolmitriptan
Moxifloxacin	

Index

Order Form

Current Clinical Strategies books can also be purchased at all medical bookstores

Title	Book	CD
Treatment Guidelines in Medicine, 2006 Edition	$19.95	$36.95
Psychiatry History Taking, Third Edition	$12.95	$28.95
Psychiatry, 2006 Edition	$12.95	$28.95
Pediatric Drug Reference, 2004 Edition	$9.95	$28.95
Anesthesiology, 2004-2005 Edition	$16.95	$28.95
Medicine, 2005 Edition	$16.95	$28.95
Pediatric Treatment Guidelines, 2004 Edition	$19.95	$29.95
Physician's Drug Manual, 2005 Edition	$9.95	$28.95
Surgery, Sixth Edition	$12.95	$28.95
Gynecology and Obstetrics, 2006 Edition	$16.95	$30.95
Pediatrics, 2004 Edition	$12.95	$28.95
Family Medicine, 2006 Edition	$26.95	$46.95
History and Physical Examination in Medicine, Tenth Edition	$14.95	$28.95
Outpatient and Primary Care Medicine, 2005 Edition	$16.95	$28.95
Critical Care Medicine, 2005 Edition	$16.95	$32.95
Handbook of Psychiatric Drugs, 2005 Edition	$12.95	$28.95
Pediatric History and Physical Examination, Fourth Edition	$12.95	$28.95
Current Clinical Strategies CD-ROM Collection for Palm, Pocket PC, Windows, and Macintosh		$49.95

CD-ROMs are compatible with Palm, Pocket PC, Windows and Macintosh.

Quan-tity	Title	Amount

Order by Phone: 800-331-8227 or 949-348-8404
Fax: 800-965-9420 or 949-348-8405
Internet Orders: http://www.ccspublishing.com/ccs
Mail Orders:

Current Clinical Strategies Publishing
27071 Cabot Road, Suite 126
Laguna Hills, California 92653

Credit Card Number: _____

Exp: ____/____

A shipping charge of $5.00 will be added to each order

Signature: _____

Check Enclosed _____

Phone Number: (_____)_____

Name and Address (please print):

_____

_____

_____

_____

3533